European School of Oncology

Monographs

Series Editor: U. Veronesi

J.C. Holland R. Zittoun (Eds.)

Psychosocial Aspects of Oncology

Springer-Verlag Berlin Heidelberg NewYork
London Paris Tokyo Hong Kong

Jimmie C. Holland

Psychiatry Service
Memorial Sloan-Kettering Cancer Center
1275 York Avenue
New York, N.Y. 10021, USA

Robert Zittoun

Service d'Hématologie
Hôtel-Dieu
1, place du Parvis Notre Dame
75181 Paris Cedex 04, France

The European School of Oncology gratefully acknowledges sponsorship for the Psychosocial Aspects of Oncology Task Force received from the Upjohn Company, developers of Alprazolam (Xanax™ tablets) and Triazolam (Halcion™ tablets).

ISBN-13: 978-3-642-46697-7 e-ISBN-13: 978-3-642-46695-3
DOI: 10.1007/978-3-642-46695-3

Library of Congress Cataloging-in-Publication Data
Psychosocial aspects of oncology / J. C. Holland, R. Zittoun (eds.). p. cm.–(Monographs / European School of Oncology) "The European School of Oncology gratefully acknowledges sponsorship for the Psychosocial Aspects of Oncology Task Force..."–T.p. verso. Includes bibliographical references.

1. Cancer–Psychological aspects. 2. Cancer–Social aspects. 3. Oncology–Philosophy. I. Holland, Jimmie C. II. Zittoun, R. III. European School of Oncology. Psychosocial Aspects of Oncology Task Force. IV. Series: Monographs (European School of Oncology) [DNLM: 1. Neoplasms–psychology. QZ 200 P9748] RC262.P783 1990 616.99'4'0019–dc20 DNLM/DLC for Library of Congress 90-9469 CIP

2123/3145-543210 – Printed on acid-free paper

Foreword

The European School of Oncology came into existence to respond to a need for information, education and training in the field of the diagnosis and treatment of cancer. There are two main reasons why such an initiative was considered necessary. Firstly, the teaching of oncology requires a rigorously multidisciplinary approach which is difficult for the Universities to put into practice since their system is mainly disciplinary orientated. Secondly, the rate of technological development that impinges on the diagnosis and treatment of cancer has been so rapid that it is not an easy task for medical faculties to adapt their curricula flexibly.

With its residential courses for organ pathologies and the seminars on new techniques (laser, monoclonal antibodies, imaging techniques etc.) or on the principal therapeutic controversies (conservative or mutilating surgery, primary or adjuvant chemotherapy, radiotherapy alone or integrated), it is the ambition of the European School of Oncology to fill a cultural and scientific gap and, thereby, create a bridge between the University and Industry and between these two and daily medical practice.

One of the more recent initiatives of ESO has been the institution of permanent study groups, also called task forces, where a limited number of leading experts are invited to meet once a year with the aim of defining the state of the art and possibly reaching a consensus on future developments in specific fields of oncology.

The ESO Monograph series was designed with the specific purpose of disseminating the results of these study group meetings, and providing concise and updated reviews of the topic discussed.

It was decided to keep the layout relatively simple, in order to restrict the costs and make the monographs available in the shortest possible time, thus overcoming a common problem in medical literature: that of the material being outdated even before publication.

Umberto Veronesi
Chairman, Scientific Committee
European School of Oncology

Contents

I. Historical Overview

Psychosocial Issues in Oncology: A Historical Perspective

Jimmie C. Holland [1], Robert Zittoun [2]

1 Psychiatry Service, Memorial Sloan-Kettering Cancer Center, 1275 York Avenue, New York, NY 10021, USA
2 Service d'Hématologie, Hôtel Dieu, 1, Place du Parvis Notre Dame, Paris 75181 Cedex 04, France

An understanding of the psychosocial problems that cancer patients and their families face must take into account not only the actual manifestations of the disease, but the *meaning* individuals attach to it. Known as a global scourge, cancer has remained the most feared disease among all societies. It has also, across cultures, been the single disease considered so frightening that physicians protected the patient from knowledge of the diagnosis. The reasons for these perceptions are understandable. No treatment existed until surgery provided the first curative treatment of cancer, after general anaesthesia came into use about the middle of the nineteenth century. Even then, cure was extremely rare. "Cancer equals death" was indeed largely true. Control of pain and distressing symptoms associated with the advanced stages of disease was also poor. The dread and fear attached to cancer came from the perception that it sentenced one to a painful death.

Cancer Treatment and Attitudes: 1850-1950

In comparing reactions to cancer and other diseases, heart disease never aroused the same sense of horror and fear as cancer. The diagnosis also caused the person and the family to feel stigmatised, isolated and humiliated [1]. The patient felt especially isolated since the family and physician shared the truth of the diagnosis while maintaining the charade of a minor illness with the patient. In *The Death of Ivan Ilyich*, Tolstoy provides a poignant literary example of how Ivan Ilyich, in nineteenth-century Russia, recognised his fatal disease while those around him maintained a pretense that he was scarcely ill, except his devoted servant who comforted him by his honest acknowledgement of his condition [2].

In those early days, the rare possibility of cure depended on early diagnosis of localised disease which could be fully removed by surgery. For the first time it became important to change the public perception. The first cancer education began in Europe in the 1890s, when Winter, a gynaecologist in East Prussia, urged women to be better informed about the danger signals of cancer. They were particularly at risk of not seeking help out of modesty and shame. A newspaper campaign in East and West Prussia in 1903 publicised the early warning signs of cancer. Childe began a similar campaign in England to educate and inform the public that cancer, when diagnosed early, was not a death warrant; early cancer *could* be cured by surgery. Childe also advocated the establishment of national cancer control societies worldwide to create a more informed public [3]. The American Society for Control of Cancer was formed in 1913. Later renamed the American Cancer Society, it was set up to counter the ignorance and fears by disseminating knowledge of the symptoms, treatment and prevention of cancer. A special Women's Field Army was developed to teach women, as in Europe, about early symptoms of breast and uterine cancer and reduce the reluctance to consult a physician for gynaecological problems. Physicians also needed education to counter their pessimism, which led them to tell patients not to seek treatment for cancer [4].

During the nineteenth century, most patients with cancer were managed by their families.

Others were cared for in facilities provided by compassionate sisters with support from the church, representing the beginnings of the hospice movement in Europe: the hospice "Dames du Calvaire", founded by Jeanne Garnier in Paris, was followed by the St. Joseph Hospice in Dublin, where Cecily Saunders worked before starting the St. Christopher's Hospice. Many concepts of humanistic and comfort care have early roots in these homes for people dying with cancer.

The development of radiotherapy in the early part of the twentieth century added a new treatment for cancer. The first Radium Institute was established in Paris in 1909, and it was followed rapidly by others around the world. Initially, radiation largely offered only palliation after surgical failure and the dose could not be quantitated, often causing burns and painful side effects [5]. The curative effects began to be demonstrated in the 1920s with the ability to control the dose.

By the 1930s, cancer began to receive wider attention from the medical research community. The International Union Against Cancer (UICC) was formed, bringing together the several national cancer societies in existence. The National Cancer Institute in the United States was established in 1937 and provided the first model for government-supported biomedical cancer research. Until then, basic research in cancer biology had been limited.

Treatment and Attitudes: 1950 - 1975

The development of the first anticancer agent added chemotherapy to cancer treatment in the early 1950s. The first responses of acute leukaemia to nitrogen mustard, a drug that was developed from World War II research on war gases, were seen, and the first cure of a cancer, choriocarcinoma, by a single chemotherapeutic agent, methotrexate, was achieved at about the same time [6]. The successful treatment of Hodgkin's disease, childhood leukaemia and testicular cancer by drugs opened a new era [7]. The development of the medical subspecialities haematology and oncology, and their paediatric counterparts, provided new opportunities for continuity of care, psychosocial support and greater attention to supportive and palliative care. Paediatric oncology was attuned to psychosocial issues, well in advance of those dealing with adults. Nicole Alby in Paris and Lansky in the United States stand out as early psychosocial researchers in childhood cancer who applied their expertise to children's care.

Psychosocial support also began to increase for cancer patients in the 1950s. In the United States, the training of social workers for assistance of patients with cancer provided the first professional discipline devoted to care of these issues in cancer. They were highly effective, joining the physician and nurse in the new concept of a health care team. In fact, some of the early observations about cancer were reported by Ruth Abrams in Boston, working at the Massachusetts General Hospital [8].

As more extensive (and more often curative) surgical treatments developed, such as laryngectomy and colostomy, surgeons began to ask former patients who had had the procedure to speak with patients anticipating similar surgery. This was often critical in encouraging the person to consent to radical procedures leading to loss of voice or normal bowel function, even when known to be curative. Laryngectomy and Ostomy Clubs, as well as a Cured Cancer Club for patients cured of cancer, developed in the United States. They helped patients face the severe stigma and prejudices that existed at that time against one who had had cancer. Also, support for cancer patients was increased through the American Cancer Society's Field and Service programmes. These programmes provided patients with supplies, such as bandages and transportation, and volunteers provided information and counselling to cancer patients and their families.

Psychological support for women who had had breast cancer was developed by Teresa Lasser and Fannie Rosenau in New York in the 1950s. Both had undergone a mastectomy and experienced the profound isolation and distress which could not be discussed with others. The impact of their efforts was particularly significant, occurring as it did at a time when mention of either cancer or the sexual organs was taboo in polite society and in the news media. Their postmastectomy support programme, called Reach-to-Recovery, based on the arm exercise as a metaphor for recovery, was taken over by the American Cancer Society. The programme's worldwide expansion has provided a highly successful self-help resource for mastectomy patients. There are Reach-for-Recovery organisations in most countries now which are widely accepted by physicians as an aid in their patients' psychological adjustment.

Despite wide endorsement by patients, these organisations fought an uphill battle to gain acceptance by the medical community. Physicians were slow to acknowledge that there was a unique role for patients to support and encourage others with the same diagnosis and treatment. They feared inappropriate advice and intrusion on the doctor-patient relationship. Peer support has been most readily accepted in the United States because of the widely accepted use of approaches such as Alcoholics Anonymous.

Psychiatrists and psychologists made several contributions to cancer that added concern for patients' quality of life. First, they described the adaptation of patients to cancer, noting the change in pattern of communication with advancing illness and the prominence of guilt as a reaction [8,9]. Second, the group at Memorial Hospital in New York offered the first description of the reactions of patients to the extensive physical and functional changes caused by colostomy and radical mastectomy [10,11]. Third, in both Europe and the United States the interest in psychosomatic medicine led many psychiatrists to seek psychodynamic explanations for vulnerability to cancer, though studies were based on retrospective and anecdotal evidence [12]. Psychiatrists in the United States also offered new insights into individuals' responses to hearing the diagnosis of cancer, into facing and discussing death and into coping with disease [13,14].

Fourth, and important for care of the fatally ill with cancer, was the development of concern for the psychosocial aspects of patients facing death. The hospice movement in Europe increased the attention for the quality of life and control of symptoms of dying patients. Cecily Saunders and the group at St. Christopher's Hospice in London spread their concepts of care to other countries. In 1970, the first hospice was opened in the United States. Kübler-Ross, a Swiss-born American psychiatrist, did much to improve communication with the dying cancer patient [15]. Her work brought out the tendency of staff to avoid discussions of impending death with the patient. She also noted the problems of society in facing death, which was a taboo topic. Her work started the thanatology movement in the United States. Loma Feigenberg, a psychiatrist at the Karolinska Radiumhemmet for many years, also made important contributions to the understanding of reactions to dying. He encouraged international efforts in this direction by the formation of the International Study Group on Dying, which is still an active and viable group.

Fifth, and of great importance, has been the role of mental health professionals in encouraging greater candour about revealing the diagnosis of cancer. The debates began in the United States in the 1950s about the questionable wisdom of never revealing the diagnosis of cancer. In a poll taken in 1961 by Oken [16], over 90% of physicians reported that they never told the diagnosis of cancer to the patient, revealing it only to the family. A group of psychiatrists and oncologists began to propose that more harm was being done by telling a lie, resulting in the loss of trust in the physician and impacting negatively on the honesty of the physician's interaction with the patient. Some doctors began changing their practice and found that both they and their patient were more comfortable, resulting in greater understanding and absence of pretense. Since then, the public has become well informed about cancer and its treatment, and has increasingly demanded attention to the right of patients to full information about treatment benefits, side effects and other options. In that climate, as well as patients tolerating the truth about their diagnosis far better than assumed, a similar survey in 1977 showed that 97% of doctors in the U.S. do generally inform their patients of the diagnosis [17]. Internationally, using the members of the International Psychooncology Society in 1984 to gather information about the practice of telling the diagnosis in 20 countries, it was found that in many countries the practice to withhold the diagnosis continues [18]. It is a highly emotional issue which is closely bound to the cultural expectations and which changes slowly, since both physicians and laymen contribute to the patterns. However, the trend noted in all countries studied was in the direction of more open disclosure, in part as the inevitable consequence of a more universally informed society and an increasing concern by doctors and the public about psychosocial issues. These issues of secrecy complicate the practice of obtaining informed consent for investigational trials which are gaining in use around the world.

Attitudes: 1975-Present

It is necessary to study psychosocial issues in cancer from a historical perspective since they reflect two realities at any given time: the medical reality of likelihood of survival with cancer in a particular period, and the concurrent societal attitudes. As more patients survive and are cured, there is less reason to remain secretive about the diagnosis. While issues of dying and death remain central for many patients, different psychosocial issues arise in relation to patients in whom cancer is a chronic illness, and those who are cured [19]. Each group has very different psychosocial issues requiring evaluation and interventions which are also quite different. It is in this present era of oncology that psychosocial issues are examined in this monograph: the patient under active treatment, the patient receiving palliative care, and the cured patient who carries risk of delayed side effects and has fears of recurrence.

Thus, in the past decade, the trends within society and the interest in psychosocial care of the disciplines of oncology, psychiatry, psychology, social work and nursing, have created a new and greater awareness of these aspects of quality of life. These changes relate to the increased optimism about cancer treatment; the increasing number of cancer survivors who write and speak openly about their experience; the trend toward greater knowledge and participation of patients in treatment decisions; the increased acceptance of and participation in cancer care of mental health disciplines; and the role of psychological and behavioural factors in cancer prevention. It is in this climate that the pioneer efforts in psychosocial oncology have occurred. Some highlights of the current psychosocial programmes are noted to place them in this perspective.

Several centres in Europe have contributed to the changes. The Psychosocial Unit at the Karolinska, currently under Bolund's direction, has been important, initially under Feigenberg, as mentioned above. The long and sustained activity of psychiatric consultation and research at the Royal Marsden, previously under Goldie and now under Greer, has thoughtfully brought a research perspective to emotions, attitudes and possible factors in survival. Maguire at Manchester has been active in the education of doctors in communication and psychosocial care, as has the group in Switzerland under Meerwein and now Hürny in Bern. Achte has provided both research and clinical observations in cancer over many years in Helsinki. Kerekartjko in Hamburg, Zittoun, as a haematologist in Paris, with strong interest in psychosocial issues, and DeNour and Baider in Israel, stand out for their contributions. Organisations such as Psychology and Cancer in France and the International Psychosomatic Study Group headed by Balthrush, each provided early networks, studying cancer from different but important outlooks. The British Psychosocial Oncology Group has been a significant force, holding regular meetings and publishing monographs which have been pioneering efforts in the field. German and Italian psychosocial oncology groups have also formed, bringing attention to the area, as has a group in Europe representing psychologists interested in cancer. Ventafridda's important contributions in pain control, as well as the palliative care effort under Twycross, overlap with psychosocial issues of dying patients.

Another approach that significantly shaped the field in Europe was the early efforts of van Dam and Bernheim to bring attention to the need for quality-of-life measurement to the EORTC clinical trials. Their role in bringing about the emphasis on this aspect of cancer research and their work with the World Health Organisation, resulted in the establishment of the WHO Quality of Life Research Centre in Amsterdam. Aaronson, joining van Dam in the EORTC and then the Dutch Cancer Institute, has worked out carefully validated scales for the measurement of quality of life in clinical trials, which are being widely adopted elsewhere (see chapter 11). Growing out of the network of psychosocial clinicians and researchers in the EORTC psychosocial efforts, the European Society for Psychosocial Oncology was formed in 1986. Under Zittoun as its first President, it has enhanced both research and clinical teaching in Europe by its conferences and collaborative efforts.

In the United States little support existed for psychosocial research before the National Cancer Plan was developed in 1972, which included a division whose goals were to enhance the rehabilitation and continuing care of cancer patients [20]. The first conference that brought together the handful of psychosocial researchers was held in 1975 in San Antonio [21]. In 1977, the first quality-of-life measurement in a clinical group in the U.S. was undertaken by Holland and the Psychiatry Committee of the Cancer and Leukaemia Group (CALGB) [22]. It has continued, funded by the National Cancer Institute, to study quality of life in patients under active treatment and more recently it has used the registry to study survivors. In 1978, the Psychosocial Collaborative Oncology Group (PSYCOG) was formed with Schmale as Chairman, operating under the NCI like the other clinical trials group and permitting collaboration of psychosocial researchers in several centres. It undertook a number of studies, including a useful prevalence study of psychiatric disorders, but was discontinued in 1985 [23]. The studies over almost a decade of Weisman and his group in Project Omega at the Massachusetts General Hospital stand as landmarks [24]. The NCI Clinical Centre contributed early training of physicians in humanistic aspects of cancer care [25].

The American Cancer Society, and especially its California Division, saw the need for support and encouragement of this emerging area of oncology in the early 1980s. The ACS sponsored two workshops, which produced monographs that were benchmarks, in 1982 and 1984. The first addressed the goals in education and research areas of the psychosocial field [26]. It resulted in the establishment of a national peer review committee for psychosocial and behavioural research (previously reviewed by basic scientists without social science backgrounds) and a national advisory committee. The second conference focused on research methods and problems facing their improvement [27]. Over 3 million dollars have gone to the support of these efforts by the ACS. A workshop to update research issues in the field will be held in 1990.

The Memorial Sloan-Kettering Cancer Center Psychiatry Service recognised the absence of available educational activities in this area in 1981 and organised the first symposium, held in New York in 1982. It was attended by many, including individuals from 15 different countries, emphasising the need for more such activities. At the second symposium, held in 1984, there was interest in those attending to form a network to encourage communication about clinical and research issues. The International Psychooncology Society (IPOS) was formed to meet those goals. Under an international board of directors, it has served as a source of international exchange through a newsletter, and more recently, to seek funding and encourage international training opportunities for psychosocial researchers to study in different countries and learn new clinical and research skills. Under its encouragement, the Mexican Psychooncology Society and the Japanese Psychooncology Society were formed with active leadership under Romero in Mexico in 1984 and Kawano in Japan in 1985. The Canadian Psychosocial Oncology Society has also been formed and is currently under the direction of Vachon. In 1988, the American Society for Psychiatric Oncology/AIDS was formed with Holland as its initial President, to encourage training in clinical care and research.

The New Field of Psychooncology

Thanks to the efforts of those mentioned above and many not recognised because of limitations of space, the care of patients with cancer today vigorously incorporates psychosocial care in its totality. Stigma, however, while less, still exists [28]. Research in these clinical care areas, as well as in prevention and detection, depends heavily upon psychosocial researchers. More centres that offer both clinical and research training in psychooncology, such as Memorial Sloan-Kettering, are badly needed. The field is recognised increasingly as a subspecialty of oncology with its own body of information dealing with both theory and practice [29].

Psychooncology, or psychosocial oncology, can be viewed as the area of oncology which studies the two psychological dimensions of cancer: the first dimension is the psychological impact of cancer on patients, their families and the staff who treat them; and the second dimension seeks to examine the role that psychological and behavioural factors may play in cancer risk and survival [30]. Prevention clearly depends on ways to alter behaviour (e.g., smoking). The new area ofpsychoneuroimmunology may provide important information about the role emotions may play in cancer aetiology and growth by some as yet unidentified change in the internal milieu. The concurrent study of emotions, en docrine and immune function in cancer patients will be important.

This monograph attempts to make the present state of information available to the practicing oncologist, giving him or her both the practical interventions for use at the bedside, and the information to assist in the recognition of the forms of distress and the range of treatments that have been shown to be effective. This first seminar given by the European School of Oncology on this topic, and the accompanying monograph, are both evidence of the degree to which the field has matured and the importance that is now being placed upon the dimension of patient care identified as psychosocial.

REFERENCES

1 Holland JC: Psychologic aspects of cancer. In: Holland JF and Frei E III (eds) Cancer Medicine. Lea & Febiger, Philadelphia 1982 pp 1175-1203, 2325-2331
2 Tolstoy L: The death of Ivan Ilyich. In: Maude L and A (trans) Great Short Works of Leo Tolstoy. Harper & Row, New York 1967 (original work published 1886)
3 American Cancer Society: Fact Book for the Medical and Related Professionals. Author, New York 1980
4 Wainwright JM: The reduction of cancer mortality. New York Med J 1911 (94):1165-1168
5 Shimkin M: Contrary to Nature. US Dept of Health and Human Services, Public Health Service. National Institutes of Health, NIH publication No 76-7291977. Washington DC 1977
6 De Vita VT, Oliverio VT, Muggia FM, Wiernik PW, Ziegler J, Goldin A, Rubin D, Henney J and Schepartz S: The drug development and clinical trials programs of the Division of Cancer Treatment, National Cancer Institute. Cancer Clin Trials 1979 (2):195-216
7 Hammond D: Progress in the study, treatment and cure of the cancers of children. In: Burchenal JH and Oettgen HF (eds) Cancer: Achievements, Challenges and Prospects for the 1980s. Vol 2. Grune & Stratton, New York 1981 pp 171-190
8 Abrams RD and Finesinger JE: Guilt reactions in patients with cancer. Cancer 1953 (6):474-483
9 Shands HC, Finesinger JE, Cobb S and Abrams RD: Psychological mechanisms in patients with cancer. Cancer 1951 (4):1159-1170
10 Sutherland AM, Orbach CE, Dyk RB and Bard M: The psychological impact of cancer and cancer surgery. I. Adaptation to the dry colostomy; preliminary report and summary of findings. Cancer 1952 (5):857-872
11 Bard M, Sutherland AM: Psychological impact of cancer and its treatment. IV. Adaptation to radical mastectomy. Cancer 1955 (8):656-672
12 Lipowski ZJ: Holistic-medical foundations of American psychiatry: A bicentennial. Am J Psychiatry 1981 (138):888-895
13 Eissler KR: The Psychiatrist and the Dying Patient. International Universities Press, New York 1955
14 Norton J: Treatment of a dying patient. Psychoanalytical Study of the Child 1963 (18):541-560
15 Kubler-Ross E: On Death and Dying. MacMillan, New York 1969
16 Oken D: What to tell cancer patients: A study of medical attitudes. JAMA 1961 (175):1120-1128
17 Novack DH, Plumer R, Smith RL, Ochitill H, Morrow GR and Bennet JM: Changes in physicians' attitudes toward telling the cancer patient. JAMA 1979 (241):897-900
18 Holland JC, Geary N, Marchini A and Tross S: An international survey of physician attitudes and practice in regard to revealing the diagnosis of cancer. Cancer Investigation 1987 (5):151-154
19 Koocher G and O'Malley J: The Damocles Syndrome. McGraw Hill, New York 1981
20 Burke LD: A national planning program for cancer rehabilitation. In: Burchenal J and Oettgen HF (eds) Cancer: Achievements, Challenges, and Prospects for the 1980s. Vol 2. Grune & Stratton, New York 1981 pp 771-791
21 Cullen JW, Fox BH and Isom RN (eds) Cancer: The Behavioural Dimensions (DHEW Publ No (NIH) 76-1074). NCI, Washington 1976
22 Holland JC, Silberfarb P, Tross S and Cella D: Psychosocial research in cancer: The Cancer and Leukemia Group B (CALGB) experience. International Congress Series Vol 702. Assessment of Quality of Life and Cancer Treatment: Proceedings of the International Workshop on Quality of Life Assessment and Cancer Treatment, Milan 11-13 December 1985. Elsevier, New York 1986 pp 89-101
23 Derogatis LR, Morrow GR, Fetting J et al: The prevalence of psychiatric disorders among cancer patients. JAMA 1983 (249):751-757
24 Weisman AD: On Dying and Denying: A Psychiatric Study of Terminality. Behavioral Publications, New York 1972
25 Artiss LK and Levine AS: Doctor-patient relation in severe illness: A seminar for oncology fellows. N Engl J Med 1973 (288):1210-1214
26 American Cancer Society Working Conference: The psychological, social, and behavioral medicine aspects of cancer: Research and professional education needs and directions for the 1980s. Cancer 1982 (50 Suppl):1919-1978
27 American Cancer Society Workshop Conference: Methodology in behavioral and psychosocial cancer research. Cancer 1984 (53 Suppl):2217-2384
28 Sontag S: Illness as Metaphor. Farrar, Straus and Giroux, New York 1977
29 Holland JC and Rowland JH (eds) Handbook of Psychooncology. Oxford University Press, Oxford 1989
30 Doll R and Peto R: The Causes of Cancer. Quantitative Estimates of Avoidable Risks of Cancer in the United States Today. Oxford University Press, Oxford 1981

II. Patient Care Issues

Crisis and Coping - Learning to Live with Cancer

Christina Bolund

Psychosocial Unit, Department of Oncology, Karolinska Hospital, S-104 01 Stockholm, Sweden

Cancer as a Personal Disaster

"If I get cancer, I would commit suicide", is a common saying not only among lay people. Professionals too, doctors and nurses, have a pessimistic outlook on cancer, not so much with respect to prognosis, but rather when it comes to enduring and mastering all those threats to personal well-being and normal existence that are connected with cancer. There is only one disease, AIDS, that has a similar strong attribution of dread. Nowadays, you may hear patients say: "Getting cancer is like being contagious with AIDS", thereby implying the strong cultural burden of symbolic evil and shame that cancer has in our culture [1].

The neoplastic diseases are not only serious and chronic diseases similar to other illnesses, they stand as symbols for the unknown and dangerous, for suffering and pain, for guilt and shame, for isolation and abandonment, for chaos and anxiety. This heavy cultural burden on cancer forms the impetus for the strong emotional reactions following the message of cancer, strong and universal enough to merit the term *crisis*. Crisis can be seen as the process - the time-bound reactions - that marks the transition from being healthy to the new life, a life of illness and constant threat. It deals with a transition period, but is also a transition of the psychology of the individual, a learning process aiming at integrating the realities and finding ways of *coping*. Coping includes all means of tackling the realities and managing to live with them with the least possible mental derangement and suffering.

The cultural burden on cancer is one explanation for the demand so often heard these days for immediate and intense psychosocial support measures for cancer patients and their relatives. It is as if the healthy person's inability to cope with the thought of getting cancer brings about a societal response: professional intervention as early as possible! However, the experience of those working in cancer care reveals a completely different picture: patients mostly do well, seem to find hidden resources of strength in themselves and in their close friends and relatives. The trauma may, however, be extremely challenging, due to the special significance of the event in the history of the individual. Falling ill with cancer often coincides with some other trauma like bereavement, children moving out, retirement. Multiple traumata constitute one of the reasons for the need of professional therapeutic help in the early stages of cancer. The need may also originate in the vulnerable personality of the patient, who reacts with mental symptoms to the strain of cancer.

The majority of patients manage without specific psychosocial interventions, whereas a minority will at some stage of the disease display psychological symptoms or distress [2,3] and will need and make use of psychiatric and/or psychotherapeutic interventions when such are available [4,5]. This phenomenon may reflect a balance between availability and demand. It may also point to the existence of an ideal balance of sources of strength: the patients' own resources, support from their close ones, communication with ordinary staff and, as a last resource, specialised psychosocial expertise.

That patients mostly manage to live through their disease does not mean that it is an easy endeavour. The route through crisis is painful and dangerous and a patient may run into blind alleys, i.e., psychological locking and crippling. Knowing the "normal psychology" of crisis and coping can help us to meet patients in a congenial way, can guide the organisation of health care and constitute a basic knowledge bank, useful when it comes to being observant of the deviations from a supposedly "normal pattern" and to intervening with patients in distress. It is important that we consider the "normal psychology" as a theoretical construct, even if based on clinical experience - *no one is normal* and every individual has his strengths and weaknesses. We will use the concepts of *crisis* and *coping* as tools to look at everyday situations in cancer care with the aim of discerning the challenges and the critical passages that cancer patients must go through. Concepts and structures are needed for any kind of knowledge and information. Psychosocial oncology is a young science, which means that its concepts and principles are not yet fully established. That is, any concept can be questioned as to its relevance. This field is a meeting place for different "schools of psychology" that use different languages. We will see how these different frames of reference may help us to discern relevant aspects of "living with cancer" rather than experiencing competition between the different schools. The introduction of crisis and coping as concepts will also introduce two relevant psychological systems, that of psychodynamic psychology and that of behavioural psychology. These will give us structures to describe clinical experience and provide frames of reference for relevant research directions.

Crisis as the Process of Learning to Live with Cancer

The first year or two following the diagnosis of cancer can be seen as a learning period and a process of adaptation, involving adjustment to uncertainty, anxiety, dependence on medical care, loss of and changes in bodily functions and roles. This learning or transition does not proceed easily; it goes with much mental pain and high costs of mental energy [5]. The crisis concept was created for reactions to all kinds of traumata [6-8], not especially for cancer, but can be adopted and transformed to cover the specific features of crisis in relation to cancer. The crisis of cancer is an existential crisis, marked by the threat to life, the closeness to medical care and the impact of changing body image and functions [9]. The loss of the illusion of immortality and omnipotence was seen by Weisman as the core of the existential plight in cancer [10]. The existential significance of cancer can be seen in the four dimensions termed by Yalom: Time, Life-Death Matters, Identity and Meaning of Life [11]. The work by Bard, partly in cancer, partly in victimology, has demonstrated clearly the similarities in reactions to cancer and to violence and crime as reactions to the loss of illusions of security and control [12].
This is illustrated in Figure 1 by the deep dip in the crisis curve.
The phases of the crisis can be described by the four stages: Shock, Reaction, Work Through and Reorientation [8].

Shock Phase

The impact of the diagnosis of cancer is catastrophic: The body cannot be trusted, all investments in the future have to be annulled, death is in the body. This existential impact has to be kept out of the conscience, in order not to bring about a psychotic reaction with breakdown of ego structure and coherence. Such a breakdown is sometimes seen in states of depersonalisation and derealisation in response to acute traumata. For a short while, maybe a few days, the inner world may be in a state of confusion. This mental state is characterised by keeping realities out of the mind, often with the help of so-called primitive defenses - splitting, projection, denial. Patients cannot tell what it feels like at the time, only afterwards: it feels like being in a shell of glass, being close to fainting, seeing the doctor talk but hearing nothing, feeling strange and not recognising reality. This state will disappear after some time, minutes, hours or days, restoring the sense of reality. Some patients make a conscious effort to

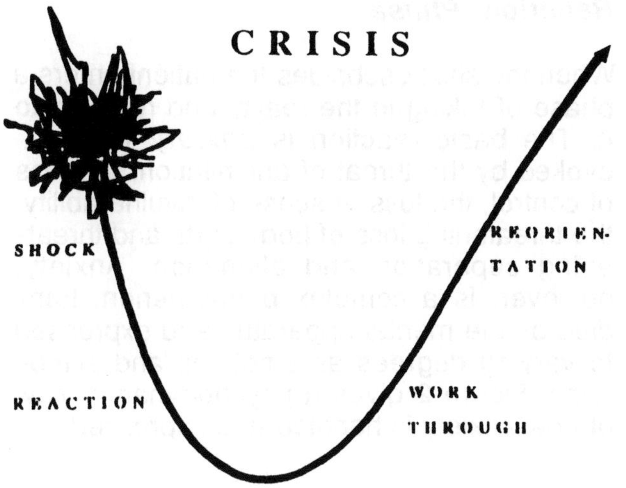

Fig. 1

grab the realities, others just notice that the strange state is over.

Very little of these dramatic reactions can be perceived by others. Instead, the communication of life-threatening diagnoses is seemingly a non-dramatic event - seldom crying or yelling, very few questions are asked, suggested procedures are hardly ever questioned. This is all in contrast to reactions in other health-care circumstances, and also in contrast to patients' behaviour at later stages of cancer treatment. The apparent lack of reactions can be understood in the light of the state of shock of the patients. It can also be understood that these reactions are necessary and self-protective and, hence, should be respected and cooperated with. This is possible in those medical situations where treatment can be started a few days later, however, in medical emergencies such as acute leukaemias and sometimes lymphomas, treatment must be instituted the same day, not leaving any time for the patient to get over the shock phase. Learning about the impact of diagnosis and the mental reactions to it has implications for the practice of how and when to tell patients. Current practice has evolved in accordance with the psychological needs of patients (and doctors?), but it would merit scrutiny and subsequent conscious choices. The varying practices of informed consent in different countries can offer a possibility to study the impact of different routines.

Clinical Implications

Empathy and intuitive understanding of these processes guide many physicians to a well-balanced sequence in the communication of the diagnosis.

This means saying what is necessary, but not too much and not too rapidly. When teaching and supervising medical students and young doctors in Stockholm in the practice of communicating "bad news", we suggest them to:

1. Let it take time, start with the results of different examinations and tests, then mention the signs of a tumour and finally arrive at the diagnosis of cancer with a brief outline of the proposed treatment.
2. Give exact and balanced information as to the danger and hope of the disease - in order to contrast the mostly pessimistic outlook on cancer that would otherwise be the patient's truth.
3. Convey also the positive messages, e.g., that the disease can be treated, that some tests are normal, thus helping the patient find a balance between good and bad, negative and positive.
4. Arrive at what will be done, "what will happen now". The important message is that the tumour can be treated . A structure for the near future is laid out - what will happen today and tomorrow. This structure is necessary to replace the chaos left by the diagnosis of cancer. This mental structure of "what will happen now" is the foremost help that we can offer; not only doctors, but also nurses and others, each providing their share of information and treatment, can help in this respect - while the relatives and friends will be there with close attention and care.
5. Split up the information to at least 2 occasions. The doctor may leave it to the nurse to repeat and expand the information. If the professionals communicate with each other, the patient may benefit from talking with a few persons, either jointly or separately.
6. A relative or friend can be invited by the patient to participate in the subsequent information session, in order to help him or her grasp the information.

7. Don't ask about emotions (!) at this early stage, it will only disturb the patient, who puts all his effort into keeping the emotions down. Practical guidelines for doctors in this dreaded part of their work are very scarse. However, an important attempt in this direction has been made by Lichter in his book Communication in Cancer Care [13].

Reaction Phase

When the shock subsides the patient enters a phase of taking in the reality and reacting to it. The basic reaction is *anxiety* (Angst), evoked by the threat of annihilation, the loss of control, the loss of sense of invulnerability, the threatening loss of body parts and threatening separation and alienation. Anxiety, however, is a complex phenomenon, handled by the mental apparatus and expressed to varying degrees as emotions and symptoms. Figure 2 gives a psychodynamic view of how anxiety is handled and expressed.

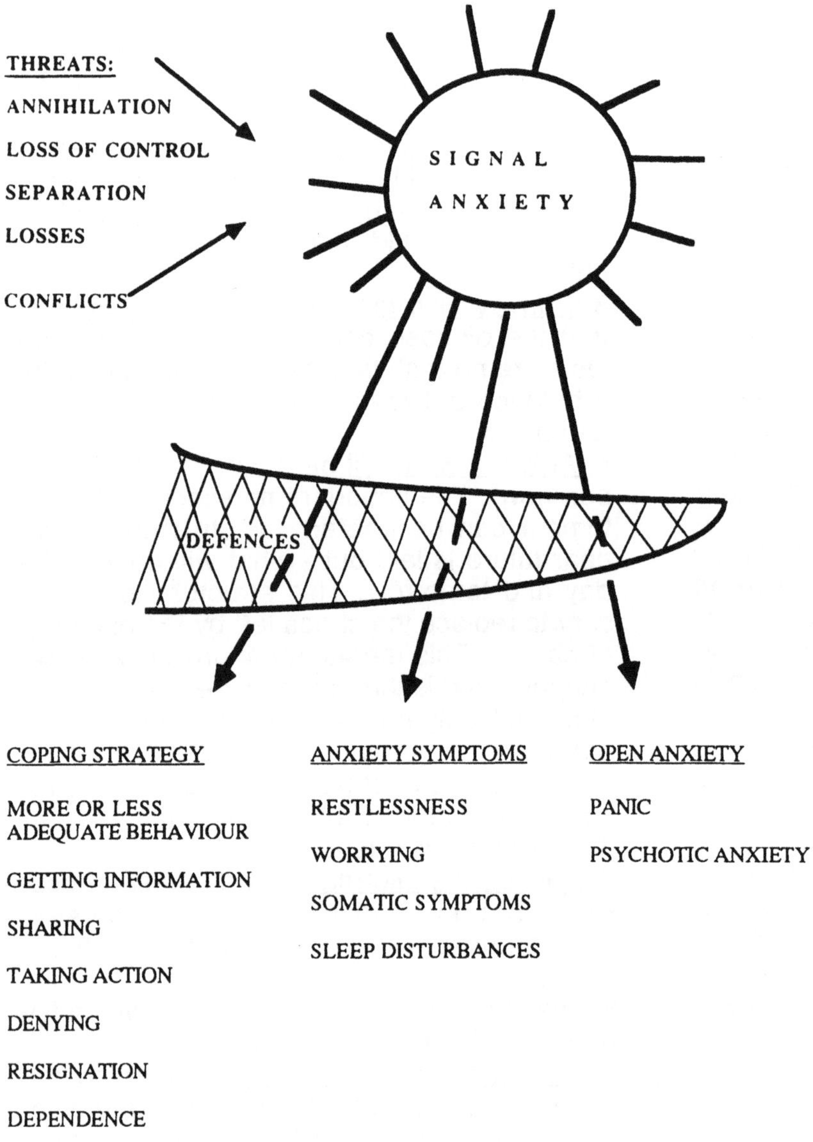

Fig. 2

What is apparent to those surrounding the patient at this stage is the consumption of energy and the defenses to anxiety. The defenses have the function of preventing that the individual be overpowered by the facts of the disease and the emotions aroused. Anxiety is the basic and strongest reaction, but also rage, bitterness and grief may be emotions too painful to bear and thus asking for defense. Defenses take on many faces. The patient may from time to time seem unaware of what has happened, "forgetting" the serious event or keeping it out of focus (examples of repression). In the verbal expressions of the patient it may be evident that he/she "knows" the diagnosis but avoids mentioning the word. Euphemisms may be used (the disease, it, the piece). The tumour may be called by name but mentioned as if it is trivial or a mistake. These are all examples of denial. There are similar defenses, working in parallel with denial: isolation (where emotions and facts are kept apart), intellectualisation, rationalisation, suppression of feelings and emotionalisation (the preoccupation with emotions without taking in real facts). Some patients can raise energy in feeling healthy, strong and happy, "better than ever", an example of reaction formation - which is close to manic defenses - sometimes turning into manic states in predisposed individuals. Projection of aggressive feelings, sadness or despair onto others is a way of starting to handle one's feelings in order to be able, at a later stage, to locate those feelings in oneself. It seems that in the crisis subsequent to a diagnosis of cancer all kinds of defenses are used in a dynamic way, including defenses that in psychiatric practice would be considered as signs of a psychotic personality structure.
Many patients go through the reaction phase with few instances and low intensity of anxiety, but the majority have some experience of anxiety symptoms at critical moments, e.g., the night before surgery, the days after the last radiation treatment was given. Patients also react with anxiety to inconsistent behaviour of doctors and staff and any other situation where confidence and security fails. Some individuals have a personality structure with inadequate defenses - expressing anxiety in the form of symptoms of worrying, restlessness, sleeping difficulties and psychosomatic symptoms of anxiety, such as palpitations, dizziness, headaches and other bodily symptoms. Rarely do you see patients with open anxiety, not at all moderated by the defenses. In those situations the patient cannot be reached by verbal contact, he will be tormented by agony, will not be helped by common anxiolytics and will require anti-psychotic doses of neuroleptics.
Regression is sometimes seen as a defense strategy - and indeed turning to the protection of others is a potent and valuable way of bearing situations that seem irresolvable and intolerable. This reaction pattern is present from early childhood and is still accessible to most adults. Moreover, health care allows regression into the patient role as a general principle. This is not always beneficial - regressive behaviour may prevent the patient from facing and solving problems - but in situations with life threat, loss of control and overwhelming lack of knowledge on the part of the patient, regression is a valuable resort and a relief of anxiety.
The mental handling of anxiety, even when successful (protection against anxiety), has a high cost of mental energy - and hence we see the patients lacking their usual resources for everyday activities and work. Or at least, the patient lacks his normal energy reserves and is let down when it comes to problems, extra activities and sexuality. Sometimes this state is interpreted as depression, which it is not. True depressive states have signs of guilt and loss of meaning, which are rare in the early stages of the cancer crisis. Patients have to be informed about the expected loss of energy in order not to feel bad and guilty for not being able to fulfil tasks that they normally would.

Clinical implications

During the reaction phase patients usually are in close contact with doctors and staff. In fact, during this phase the medical procedures force the patient to face the truth, that he/she is ill and no longer healthy. At the same time we expect and allow a great deal of regression. However, the support of patients is often inconsistent and disorganised, placing an extra burden on the patients. In

this phase adequate psychosocial attendance would involve:
1. Repeated meetings with doctor and nurse (ideally the same doctor and nurse) for continuous information and support during distressing treatments and expectancy periods. Time-consuming discussions and therapeutic talks are mostly not beneficial, not expected and limitations of time are respected by most patients. The quality, consistence and openness is of higher priority than the quantity of talking. The physician has many opportunities of helping the patient face the truth of the situation at a pace determined by the patient.
2. Mental reactions should be mentioned by the physician as an area of concern. Periodically it is in this area that the patient suffers most! Patients need to hear that these reactions are normal and not signs of mental disease, as many of them fear.
3. Areas of concern should be approached both by the doctor and the nurse, since patients will choose different areas to talk about - usually medical matters with the doctor and social concerns with the nurse.
One task is to check whether the patient has problems of such dimensions or difficulty that he/she should be offered contact with a social worker, psychologist or psychiatrist.
4. Mental preparation for transitional periods, when routines are changed, treatments instituted or stopped, hospitalisation is near its end, etc., should be given by all staff in contact with the patient. Thus, the most anxiety-provoking and distressing phases may be eased and patients will be guided towards a constructive way of setting words to problems and solving them.
5. Identity-supporting therapeutic stand means helping the patient by discussing how to solve problems, rather than solving them for him/her. In the process of discussing questions like "What would be your strategy?" ,"How do you usually act in situations like this?" one can encourage reflections on identity and personal strength, in the midst of weakness and misery.

Work Through

During the period of active medical procedures the important task is to go on, to survive as a person - both physically and mentally. It seems as though patients deal with what is necessary at that time and leave the rest to be dealt with later on, when the mental energy is no longer consumed by the task of surviving.
When the most active period of diagnostics and treatments is over, the patient is left with the hard task of understanding the new life situation and living with it. The following tasks and questions help him/her to build the puzzle of the new life:

1. Going through medical procedures gives the patient the opportunity to take in that "What has happened has happened" and is part of life. There are signs that cannot be ignored - operation scars, mutilation, loss of hair, side effects - and which tell the patient "You had a serious illness that motivated this heavy treatment. Life has changed and will not be the same again".
2. Being different is an experience that is often painful but at the same time gives insights that form a necessary basis for future life. The difference between the patient group and the staff, between patients in the hospital window and people rushing on the streets, is a painful reality - you belong to those on the weak side, no longer to those on the strong and healthy side. Being different also means being another person than before, having new experiences, having lost the innocent belief that "nothing serious can happen to me".
3. Planning for the future is a capacity most cancer patients lose for some months or years. Just the thought of next Christmas, next summer, brings forth the anxious thought: "What will have happened then? Will I be alive by that time?" As a consequence, many patients leave planning aside and live by the day, which for many is a new and uncertain way of life. Still, it gives new insights, e.g., how rich life can be when you do not put off things until tomorrow. The ability to plan is slowly regained. Often the time until the next checkup with the doctor is a time span patients dare invest in. Step by step the time that can be planned is prolonged - from weeks to months to years. Open talk about these experiences is a way of reflecting upon uncertainty and insecurity, making these anxiety-provoking phenomena conscious

and putting words to them - the first step in mastering.

4. Needing checkups is a sign of the remaining medical risk. The oncological routine of checking patients regularly for years has been questioned - Could it be that psychological problems arise just because of these regular medical visits [14]? However, the regular visits also offer a great deal of relief of letting someone else (the doctor) take the responsibility, of having the regular experience of being told "everything is fine". The regular checkups offer a possibility of splitting time into shorter periods that can be overlooked - not 10 years when anything can happen anytime, but 2 months, "in such a short time nothing can happen".

5. Worrying about symptoms is common in this phase. Any symptom or signal from the body can arouse fear of recurrence or of a new cancer. With the recent experience of learning that you have a lethal disease (mostly) without any symptoms, it is obvious that body signals cannot be trusted or understood. During this period a "hot line" to a nurse or doctor is invaluable in helping the patient learn to interpret his somatic signs again.

6. Asking "Why" is an important endeavour that many patients keep making. They turn to doctors : "Can it be that bruise, is that the cause?" "It started with that 'flue - is that to blame?" These questions help the patient look for causes. In a world where all other events have causes, only cancer is said to be a mystery, even to scientists!

The "Why" has other meanings as well: "Why me - Where is the justice?" "Why not him, that old man" - anger, jealousy and bitterness may be turned to people around.

"Why me - I always tried to tend to my health - I did not smoke or drink." As if cancer were the punishment for sins. And last, the modern meaning of "Why" is related to psychosocial causes of cancer - "Was it because daddy died, or that divorce, or those stressful weeks". It is obvious that the type of answer is changing but the need to ask is universal. The task of asking is to find structure and reason in a chaos of unpredictable events. Even guilt feelings are better to live with than experiencing life as dependent upon hazard.

7. How to use the new life is a question many patients ask themselves after having lived close to death for some time. Life is no longer taken for granted - it is questioned and valued. It may focus on relations that have been unsatisfactory - now it seems urgent to do something about them. The patient all of a sudden wants to straighten out old misunderstandings and bad habits. This often comes unexpectedly to those around and conflicts may arise with the spouse, with relatives and friends, and in the work environment. The choice of profession may be questioned, the old dream of what to dedicate your life to may be revived.

Clinical Implications

In this phase the frequent visits to the hospital have ceased and patients are often left to their own resources. If health care would take the responsibility for the rehabilitation of cancer patients much could be done in this phase:

1. A summarising talk with the physician a few months after the end of the treatment period is very useful for the patient who tries to understand what has happened and why. Patients who did not earlier have many questions now often want information on the nature of the tumour and on all aspects of treatment options, effects and side effects. It is not too late to give it now, it is needed by the patient in order to go on. A planned half-hour conversation can spare both patient and doctor much trouble.

This opportunity can also be used to judge the patient's need for special rehabilitation resources - physiotherapist, dietician, social worker, or psychotherapist.

2. Availability of a counselling telephone service is valuable for patients who have hypochondriac problems in this phase. Straightforward conversations on the nature of symptoms and how these can be handled can be seen as ways of teaching patients to cope by providing information and realistic reasoning.

3. Answering questions about "Why" not by saying yes or no, but taking the question as an invitation to talk about the thoughts and views of the patient will be very helpful in the working through of the crisis.

4. Patient groups as a means of working through are widely used in the US and Canada [15] and are currently being introduced in Europe. The experience is that a trained, professional group leader will help keeping conversations constructive and taking care of vulnerable individuals.
5. Rehabilitation programmes are scarse today [16,17] but will probably be instituted in the coming years. In cancer care, rehabilitation programmes after cancer treatment are mentioned as one of the goals for the future. Some countries have laws obliging health care to offer rehabilitation after active treatment [18].

Reorientation

The phases of the crisis are not separate in time but rather diffusely changing one into the other and they often come and go in relation to external events. Thus, the repeated checkups bring patients back into the sick role and back into the fear of detecting new manifestations of the disease. At the same time, the checkup induces a renewed work through. The relief after each checkup is a takeoff for turning to life again, leaving thoughts about the cancer and the impact of threat behind. As this is repeated many times, the patient will realise: "Here I am with a life to live." This existential notion is often bewildering - one's identity is questioned, the meaning of life is questioned, what is the life to be wished and strived for, how were life choices made before, what was wrong with my life choices before.

1. Existential questions come to the surface, are reflected upon and discussed with family members and friends. This may be experienced as a painful reappraisal of one's earlier choices and at the same time as a gift and a challenge to new insights: "Life is there with its sharp and painful questions, as in youth, when it lies in front of you." These choices and reappraisals are, however, sometimes too painful to be solved on one's own and often people in the patient's surroundings feel ill at ease and are unwilling to go into these discussions, giving the patient the feeling of being a nuisance: "Now that the treatments are over and you are healthy again, you try to complicate life unnecessarily!" Also, patients often have ambivalent feelings - on the one hand they are grateful for being alive and on the other they are dissatisfied and may be questioning themselves and others. Many patients would benefit from a talk with a professional - be it a doctor or a nurse, a therapist or a spiritual guide - to help them endure the pains and gain insights and to discuss choices.
2. Consolidating one's new identity is achieved through the repeated confrontation of one's new self (with those experiences gained) and the old situations and roles. Every time the patient goes back to any social activity: work, other professional situations, associations, church groups, circles of friends, etc., he will realise that he is not the same as before, which may be a notion that cuts both ways. Each time this happens can be seen as a small crisis that needs to be confronted, the solution of which may either reinforce or weaken the new identity.
3. The search for meaning goes on more or less consciously for most patients for some time after the disease period. The disruption of everyday life abolishes the automatic, unquestioned routines and meanings, leading to a vacuum when the critical period is over. The patient may feel lost, depressed or confused. For some patients this experience may lead to serious depression - after fighting, clinging to rational goals and efforts, keeping emotions and weakness aside, many patients have a depressive period, sometimes accelerating to depressive illness. It is not uncommon that patients will need antidepressant medication. The majority will benefit from a therapeutic contact dealing with the personal and existential aftermath of the disease period.
4. The sword of Damocles is a symbol for the experience of constantly living with the threat that "anything can happen anytime" [19]. This means that it is not only the uncertainty inherent in the cancer disease that one has to adjust to, it is rather the lost illusion of safety and control over existence that is at the core [12]. This means that former cancer patients have to put up with the existential notion that most healthy persons manage to keep unconscious: "Man is vulnerable and mortal and all human efforts to take control are futile."

Clinical Implications

1. Talks on the spiritual and philosophical aspects of illness are usually not seen as the task of health care, and health care staff often feel embarassed when they meet patients wishing to talk about these questions. It is, however, a given task for specialised psychosocial services not only to offer patients the opportunity to solve important and sometimes tormenting existential questions, but also to raise these questions in lectures, seminars and staff meetings, in order to provide a "language" for these questions in the context of health care.

2. Depression and persisting anxiety as consequences of cancer can be seen several years after the active medical procedures are over. These patients need psychiatric or psychotherapeutic assistance and would benefit from seeing a therapist experienced in cancer for a delayed crisis work through, bringing remnants of ignorance and fears of medical facts to the surface, putting the patient's reactions on the factual and realistic level - as expected and normal reactions to the past events.

These therapies are rewarding and satisfying also for the therapist who may guide a patient who has long been crippled by his emotional reactions into a state of relief, insight and functional well-being.

3. Patient groups, either professionally led or self-help groups, have much to offer the patient confronting his or her "new life". In this context they meet people who have had the same experiences and who are willing to discuss difficult questions. For months and years a peer group may be the most important support and the forum for working on important problems associated with turning to life again. The process of leaving the sick role and returning to normal life is parallelled by the ambivalence of whether to stay in the group or leave it. Leaving the group means closing the disease life and marking the definite orientation towards normal life.

Survivorship

The problems that survivors have to cope with are not new phenomenona. For generations people have survived cancer after curative surgery and/or radiotherapy. The price consisted often of mutilations and progressive scarring due to tissue-damaging radiotherapy, the effects of treatment sometimes being extremely crippling, especially in the case of growth retardation or intellectual deficiencies in young patients.

Nowadays, mutilation and radiation sequelae are reduced to a minimum by improved technical equipment and the use of combined treatments of surgery, radiotherapy and chemotherapy. Today, patients with lymphomas, testicular carcinoma, leukaemia and childhood malignancies of different types can be rescued by intensive chemotherapy in combination with surgery, bone marrow transplantation and radiotherapy. We now see new problems and strains - the prolonged treatment periods implying disruption of social contexts, severe toxicity during treatments, dramatic procedures such as bone marrow transplantation requiring long periods of hospitalisation, physiological sequelae such as decreased fertility [20]. All these interventions and sequelae lead to repercussions and demands for adjustment and adaptation.

Contrary to the expectations of many, however, the overall adjustment and quality of life of patients has not changed markedly with the more aggressive procedures. The incidence of considerable somatic side effects and mental suffering after treatment involving bone marrow transplantation is 10-25% [21,22].

In studies of survivors of childhood malignancies Li [20], Koocher and O´Malley [19] and others report that:

social adjustment is found to be adequate in the vast majority of ex-patients, who complete studies and professional training, maintain jobs and manage social relationships, including marriage and sexual relations;

somatic sequelae do continue to strain a minority of patients with decreased intellectual capacity, growth retardation and diminished or abolished fertility;

psychiatric sequelae do seem to affect ex-patients. In a majority of patients they take the form of mild mental symptoms (worrying, anxiety, nervousness) whereas in a minority of patients severe symptoms occur, requiring therapeutic attention. It is the focus of psychosocial oncology to model interventions during the disease period in order to decrease mental repercussions in later life.

Psychological adjustment has many faces, since individuals are different. Some specific patterns can be discerned:
Hypochondriac problems - worrying over any body signal and any trivial affection. It is an understandable reaction: these people have learned that any trivial symptom may be the clue of life threat, and only by being in time can one's life be saved. These patients need medical contacts to help them understand the nature of signals and symptoms and may be helped by psychotherapy to re-learn interpretation of body signals and verbalising anxiety.
Fixation in the sick role may be the psychological solution chosen by some individuals, often enhanced by the family system. It may entail secondary neurotic gains of dependency.
The Damocles Syndrome is a symbol used to describe the existential threat - anything may happen anytime - an experience opening up for appreciation of each day, once the anxiety over the uncontrollable has been dealt with.
The Polyanna Ideal means the compulsory, anxiety-driven superstructure on gratitude: you must be content, you must be happy, you should not complain, you must pay back for your guilt of being chosen to live.
The One-Day-Flower-experience: heightened joy of living, increased intensity in the appetite for life is an experience gained by quite a proportion of patients, often highly valued and much regretted when it gives way to the more balanced experience of everyday life, bearing both the fantastic and the trivial, good as well as bad.

Coping - The Efforts to Live with Cancer

The process of getting cancer and learning to live with it is best covered by the concept of crisis, whereas the coping concept applies to the variety of ways that people manage to live with cancer. In clinical practice we constantly see patients put up with strains and problems that would seem to be extreme challenges to their mental equilibrium and problem solving capacities, and yet somehow they do it. The variety of individual solutions is hard to systematise, both with respect to the psychological mechanisms adopted and to the adequacy - who is in a position to judge which tactics are adequate when it comes to surviving as an individual, on individual conditions, when it is the individual who has to make it and accept the consequences.
The concept of coping has gained great popularity and diffusion [23-25] and yet the term has not been defined adequately. Lazarus and coworkers [26] have set the fundamentals of a definition and description of the functions of coping :
The cognitive dimension. In order to solve a problem situation the first task is to recognise the problems and sort them out in terms of origin and demands.
The mental dimension is fundamental in that the person has to deal with the stress, the anxiety and the emotional reactions before being able to handle the external situation. Personality factors such as defenses against anxiety, tolerance of anxiety, reality orientation, trust and ego strength affect the individual's ability to confront, endure and solve any problem.
The behavioural dimension has to do with the individual's capacity for problem solving, often modelled in childhood and reinforced in adult life.
Lazarus [26] also describes the outcome dimensions of coping: the external tasks that have to be solved and the internal equilibrium that has to be maintained. He arrives at a definition of coping: "Efforts both action-oriented and intrapsychic to manage (that is, to master, tolerate, reduce, minimise) environmental and internal demands and conflicts among them, which tax or exceed a person's resources."
A central concept in coping is control and the individual's tendency to rely on himself - internal locus of control - or upon external factors, such as chance, God, fate, or the beneficial or malevolent power of other human beings - external locus of control (after Rotter [27]). In the same tradition, the concept of learned helplessness [28] and helplessness /

hopelessness [29] is seen as a disposition towards giving up, not only the active fight for health but also by postulated neuroimmunological mechanisms impairing the physiological defense against cancer [29].
The meaning of the disease to the individual may vary greatly and will imply different coping approaches. Lipowski [30] lists 8 different and common meanings of disease in our culture: Challenge, enemy, punishment, weakness, relief, strategy, loss and value. According to Lipowski [30] the recognition of these attributions can be minimising (ignoring, denying, rationalising) or subject to vigilant focusing and leading to behaviours of tackling, capitulation, or avoidance.
Most authors look for specific patterns of coping, predicting the outcome either in psychosocial mastery or in prognosis of the cancer. By contrast, Weisman [31] gives a pragmatic description of different coping styles that patients can be seen to adopt and of which the researcher during therapeutic conversations will understand the dynamic function.
The list of coping strategies according to Weisman is unstructured but makes clinical sense:

1. Seek more information (rational inquiry);
2. Share concern and talk with others (mutuality);
3. Laugh it off (affect reversal);
4. Try to forget; put it out of your mind (suppression);
5. Do other things for distraction (displacement);
6. Take firm action (confrontation);
7. Accept but find something favourable (revision);
8. Do anything (impulsivity);
9. Submit to the inevitable (resignation);
10. Review alternatives (rational reflection);
11. Reduce tension by drinking, drugs;
12. Withdraw into isolation (escape);
13. Blame someone (externalise);
14. Seek direction (compliance);
15. Blame yourself (internalise, guilt).

In a research project the coping pattern and vulnerability of cancer patients were assessed shortly after diagnosis and these patterns were tested for their ability to predict psychosocial outcome in the course of the disease. In a later phase an intervention programme (counselling or teaching coping strategy) was instituted and tested for its possible power to prevent adjustment problems [32]. Weisman has coined the term "counter-coping" for the reactions on the part of the doctor or staff and their cooperation with the patient's coping style, in order to achieve safe conduct for the patient all through the different phases of the illness [32].
Can coping be changed by will or training? The answer to this question will depend on different notions about the roots of different styles of coping - whether they are inherent in the personality structure or learned during active life, and, hence, possible to change by relearning. The experience of Weisman and Worden was equivocal [32]. Another attempt is made by Greer and coworkers, who identify patients reacting with helplessness or stoicism to the diagnosis of breast cancer and, with the aim of improving the prognosis, employ adjuvant psychotherapy, teaching patients confrontative and fighting behaviour [33]. The outcome of this programme has to be awaited.
A dimension of coping, clinically of utmost importance both for the general well-being and the quality of life of patients, is the sense of meaning and purpose of life. This dimension has been absent from most theoretical coping concepts. However, Hinton [34] stresses the sense of fulfillment and meaning of one's life as an important factor for the mental adjustment to dying.
In the coping model of Antonovsky - the salutogenic model of health - the central concept is the "sense of coherence" [35]. This term covers the capacity to perceive the world as comprehensible, structured, manageable and meaningful. This capacity helps the individual to go through stressful events and turmoil without getting lost and without losing confidence in a meaningful world.
This model explains not only the difference between different persons with respect to their inborn sense of coherence, but the importance of structure and coherence in the outer world as a help to the person in anguish and chaos. Hence we can sense the importance of health care organisation on the gross and especially on the micro level for the welfare of vulnerable patients.

The important factors in coping should not only be seen as the strength or weakness of the individual patient but also as the adequacy of the surrounding social structure in its contribution to consistency and meaning. In times of illness the health care system is the most important structure, that upon which your health, life or death depends. If that system is not functioning in a coherent and meaningful way, confidence and security will fail and patients will be subject to chaos and anxiety much more than if the structure were trustworthy. It is the experience of psychiatrists and other psychosocial consultants that our specialised functions are only relevant if the medical care is functioning. If it is not, there is no point in psychotherapy. The best you can do for the patient then is to achieve decent and consistent treatment and care. Hence, I have worked out a dual model of coping with illness and threat, based on the patient's factors on the one hand and the health care organisation on the other:

Patient's coping factors

Ego strength and maturity
- existing and flexible defenses
- reality orientation
- regression in service of the ego

Social safety network
Continuity of social/cultural life

Health care system factors

Technical and human skills
Consistency and continuity
Adequate medical care
Attention to individual needs
Readily providing extra time and/or support when patient's own resources are failing.

It is common for us to see psychosocial endeavours purely on the individualistic level and forget about the social structure of the system that we and the patients are part of. In situations of extreme strain on individuals - patients and staff - as in care for life-threatening illness, we are dependent on routines, order, social rules and a sense of coherence and meaning. Security, order and meaning are crucial for our ability to care for the individual.

REFERENCES

1 Sontag S: Illness as a Metaphor. Farrar, Strauss and Giroux, New York 1978
2 Derogatis LR et al: The prevalence of psychiatric disorders among cancer patients. JAMA 1983 (249):751-757
3 Plumb M and Holland J: Comparative studies on psychological function in patients with advanced cancer II. Interviewer-rated current and past psychological symptoms. Psychosom Med 1981 (43):243-254
4 Capone MA, Westie KS, Chitwood JS, Feigenbaum D and Good RS: Crisis intervention: A functional model for hospitalized cancer patients. Am J Orthopsych 1979 (49):598-607
5 Greer S and Silberfarb PM: Psychological concomitants of cancer. Current state of research. Psychol Med 1982 (12):563-573
6 Caplan G: Principles of Preventive Psychiatry. Basic Books Inc, New York 1964
7 Lindemann E: Symptomatology and management of acute grief. Am J Psychiatry 1944 (101):141-148
8 Cullberg J: Crisis and Development. Bonniers, Stockholm 1975
9 Bard M and Sutherland: Psychological impact of cancer and treatment. Adaptation to radical mastectomy. Cancer 1955 (8):656-672
10 Weisman AD: The Coping Capacity. On the Nature of Being Mortal. Human Sciences Press, New York 1984
11 Yalom ID: Existential Psychotherapy. Basic Books Inc, New York 1980
12 Bard M and Sangrey D: The Crime Victim's Book. Bunner Mazel Publ. Psychosocial Stress Series VI. New York 1986
13 Lichter I: Communication in Cancer Care. Churchill Livingstone 1987
14 Jacobs C et al: Behavior of cancer patients: A randomized study of the effects of education and peer groups. Am J Clin Onc 1983 (6):347-350
15 Taylor SE et al: Social support, support groups and the cancer patient. J Cons Clin Psychol 1986 (54):608-615
16 Lehman JF et al: Cancer rehabilitation: Assessment of needs, development and evaluation of a model of care. Arch Phys Med Rehab 1977 (59):410-423
17 Heyde et al: Rehabilitation Krebskranker unter Einschluss schöpferischer Therapien. Rehabilitation 1983 (22):25-27
18 Communication from Finnish Cancer Society
19 Koocher GP and O'Malley JE: Damocles Syndrome: Psychological Consequences of Surviving Childhood Cancer. McGraw-Hill, New York 1981
20 Li FP: Follow up of survivors of childhood cancer. Cancer 1977 (39):1176-1178
21 Wolcott DL et al: Adaptation of adult bone marrow transplant recipient long-term survivors. Transplantation 1986 (4):478-484
22 Lesko LM et al: Psychosocial functioning of adult acute leukemia survivors treated with bone marrow transplantation or standars chemotherapy. Proc Ann Meet Am Soc Clin Oncol 1987 (6):A1002
23 Haan N: Coping and Defending: Processes of Self-Environment Organisation. Academic Press, New York 1977
24 Visotsky H, Hamburg D, Goss M and Lebouits B: Coping behavior under extreme stress. Arch Gen Psych 1961 (5):423-448
25 National Cancer Institute: Coping with Cancer. A Resource for the Health Professionals. US Department of Health and Human Services 1980
26 Lazarus R: Stress and coping as factors in health and illness. In: Cohen J et al (eds) Psychosocial Aspects of Cancer. Raven Press, New York 1982 pp 163-198
27 Rotter JB: Generalized expectancies for internal versus external control of reinforcement. Psychological Monographs 1966 (80)
28 Seligman MPF: Helplessness. On Depression, Development and Death. WH Freeman & Co, San Francisco 1975
29 Schmaale A: Giving up as the final common pathway to changes in health. Adv in Psychosom Med 1972 (8):20-40
30 Lipowsky ZJ: Physical illness, the individual and the coping processes. Psychiatry in Medicine 1970 (1):91-102
31 Weisman AD: Coping with Cancer. McGraw-Hill, New York 1979
32 Weisman AD and Worden W: Preventive psychosocial intervention with newly diagnosed cancer patients. Gen Hosp Psych 1984 (6):243-249
33 Watson M: The development of psychosocial interventions in oncology settings. ESPO. First meeting, Madrid 1987
34 Hinton J: The influence of previous personality on reactions to having terminal cancer. Omega 1975 (6):95-111
35 Antonovsky A: Health, Stress and Coping. Jossey-Bass Publishers1980

Patient Information and Participation

Robert Zittoun

Service d'Hématologie, Hôtel Dieu, 1, Place du Parvis Notre Dame, Paris 75181 Cedex 04, France

In the field of disease prevention and treatment, the last decades have been characterised by an increasing demand by patients and the general public for information on and participation in medical decision-making. This has resulted in a profound change in the relationship between patients and caregivers. As an example, until the1950s most physicians preferred not to reveal cancer diagnosis to their patients, whereas the opposite attitude was progressively adopted by the late 1970s [1]. Diagnosis is more easily disclosed when it concerns a form of cancer with a high probability of cure - e.g. Hodgkin's disease - but even diseases with a probable fatal outcome such as lung cancer or adult acute leukaemia are more and more commonly announced to patients [2]. Disclosure of such diagnosis in spite of poor prognosis is frequently felt by physicians as a necessity, in order to make acceptable proposed treatments with potentially severe side effects, and is also imposed as an ethical obligation if one considers enrolling the patient into a clinical trial, with duly informed consent.

The current approach must be considered within the general framework of patients as consumers, with an increasing demand by the consumers for access to information and for some control over the proposed product. It derives from the current emphasis on individual responsibility and autonomy: in addition to the human right to health and social protection, there is a more pronounced concern for the individual's right to control his/her own life and death ; therefore, the right to full medical information and participation in medical decision-making is advocated [1]. The model of the ideal patient's behaviour and of the ideal patient-physician relationship has profoundly changed: patients are no longer viewed as passive objects of care following full transfer of responsibility to a conscientious physician - paternalistic/compliance model; they are nowadays considered as equally sharing responsibility in treatment choices, even if one takes into account the uncertainty inherent in medical decision-making - contractual/participation model [3-5].

Patient participation in (cancer) care must be viewed within the general framework of contemporary patient/physician interaction: physicians diagnose and treat *diseases* , i.e., abnormalities in the structure and function of body organs and systems, whereas patients suffer from *illnesses* - difficulties of living resulting from sickness. Both concepts and attitudes are culturally influenced [6]. Patient participation depends on the interaction between the two models.

In the present section, the following aspects of patient participation will be discussed: possible benefits and drawbacks, factors interfering with patients' quest for participation and patient preferences, distinction between various types of participation, and, finally, the different ways to improve participation in these conditions.

Potential Benefits of Patient Participation

Patient Participation Corresponds to an Ethical Obligation and a Social Demand

The present state of democracy reached in our Western countries has resulted in a demand for more equality and individual autonomy, especially among members of socially subordinate groups [3]. Informed consent in medical decisions is not only a prerequisite for enrolling patients in clinical trials, according to the Helsinki rules, but is also felt as a necessity before treating patients according to well proven methods. Physicians are less easily accepted as parent-like beings exercising unilateral authority on the basis of incommunicable knowledge; the wave of consumerism has encouraged patients to seek information and to preserve their feelings of individuality and autonomy and their sense of personal dignity by active participation in the medical decision-making process [4]. The social demand, through groups, self-help movements, the media and sometimes lawyers in the case of conflict about the final result of a decision, has led governments and administrations to publish rules and recommendations on the patient's rights. The Patient's Bill of Rights published by the American Hospital Association states that patients should not only participate in medical decision-making but also have higher authority than physicians in certain situations concerning themselves.

Patient Participation Represents a Therapeutic Objective

It has been postulated that the results of treatment, e.g., response rate and survival, could be improved by active patient participation. This assumption corresponds to a frequent hope in the patient's mind that active participation could increase the chances of cure. Although a few studies have provided some evidence of a significant relationship between patient orientation and treatment results in diseases like hypertension [7], no such relationship has been shown so far in malignancies. However, patient participation can have several beneficial effects, e.g.:

- ensuring better adaptation of the medical decision to a patient's individual needs and preferences, thereby enabling caregivers to provide more satisfactory care;
- improving patients' compliance with treatment, since the treatment choice has resulted from their own participation in the medical decision;
- decreasing the risk of side effects, as patients are more aware and able to evaluate medical intervention in terms of cost, inconvenience, discomfort and dysfunction [8];
- decreasing the level of anxiety and depression and helping patients cope with their disease;
- restoring patients' self-esteem and self-reliance;
- improving the quality of life of patients during and after completion of treatment. In fact, enriching the quality of life could be independent from the quality of adjustment to decisions made: giving people the opportunity to take responsibility for decisions which affect their lives is considered beneficial *per se*, improving self-esteem, mental health and therefore the participant's quality of life [9].

Several recent studies have begun to confirm these expected benefits from patient participation: psychological preparation in an early phase of physician-patient interaction was found helpful in patients with seminomatous testicular cancer, improving satisfaction with interpersonal and sexual relationships in spite of the important limitations resulting from disease and treatment [10]. In their study of 30 patients with early breast cancer, Morris and Royle have observed a significantly higher percentage of pre- and post-operative anxiety and depression in patients not offered the choice between mastectomy and lumpectomy plus radiotherapy; they conclude that with proper counselling patients suffer less stress if they are allowed to take an active part in the treatment of their cancer [11]. Another study has shown less side-effects such as nausea, vomiting, poor appetite and alopecia, and better quality of life and satisfaction when patients with advanced cancer were allowed to choose between two different chemotherapy regimens - e.g., doxorubicin versus mitozantrone - following a first allocation in a randomised cross-over study [8].

Conversely, disadvantages and risks of poor patient participation have been repeatedly underlined, whether the caregivers or the patients are primarily responsible for this poor participation. Kleinman et al. have observed that the failure to directly elicit patients' attitudes and desires about their care can have devastating effects on therapeutic success [6]. Treatments selected without patient participation could be misunderstood, with increased risk of poor compliance or reactive depression. Loss of decision-making power could be the heaviest blow to the patients' morale [12], and non-compliance may represent a patient's attempt to gain some control over treatment [13,14]. The question could even be raised whether the search of many patients for alternative therapies could be a way of keeping some power in the face of an overpowerful medical science.

Participation Helps Patients to Cope with their Disease

Coping is generally viewed as a psychological reaction to stress and other negative consequences of cancer. It results in various behaviours determined by active psychological involvement in the face of adversity. According to some popular thinking, fighting their own cancers by positive attitudes and concrete action could help patients achieve remission and cure. More realistically, obtaining information and participating in the medical decision-making process and one's own care represents an important part of coping strategies and can help to reduce anxiety and psychological distress [11].

However, one should avoid an oversimplistic view of equating coping with maximum information and participation: individuals do better when the intensity of the information they receive is consistent with their coping strategy. There is a range of differences between information seekers and information avoiders [4]. Adaptation mechanisms regularly include denial to some extent, and anxiety may result from an excess of information. It has been observed that information seekers may experience both more satisfaction and more distress from their involvement in medical knowledge and decision-making [4]. In addition, a sense of urgency about the need to make a treatment decision may create enormous stress rather than engaging the patient in rationalisation and confidence [5]. On the other hand, the desire of some patients for participation is minimal, especially in information avoiders, for whom denial is an essential part of their coping strategy, or for some when disease results in reduced physical and psychosocial capacities. Information and participation are included in the coping process, but they must be modulated according to patients personalities, situations and needs.

Possible Pitfalls and Limitations of Patient Participation

Patients' Ambivalence

The problem of participation, especially in medical decision-making, must always be viewed while taking into account the patient's permanent ambivalence. Cancer severely affects the psychosocial equilibrium - "economy" - of the patient, by revealing a real risk of death, equivalent to an absolute loss of power. As a result, the patient will try:

- to maintain or restore his/her own power, by collecting a maximum of information and making his/her own choices;
- to delegate his/her power to the physicians, nurses and other caregivers. When a physician, with the ethical and therapeutic concerns mentioned earlier, wants to let the final decision be made by the patient, following complete information on the treatment alternatives, the frequent answer is: "You are the doctor, it's up to you to decide". In a study by Strull et al., less than one-fourth of the patients wished to make joint decisions with the clinicians, although sharing decision-making had been advocated as ideal [15].

Disease and Regression

Regression is a common psychoanalytic concept defined by the return to an earlier stage of psychological development, with a possible resurgence of archaic forms of thinking, relationships to objects, and behaviour. This can correspond, according to the Freudian theory on sexuality, to lateral ways of satisfaction [16]. In the case of severe somatic disease, regression is generally viewed as a primitive psychic structure, with consequent infantile dependence behaviour. Patients appreciate some degree of dependence and look for an authority figure who will allow them to get rid of their own responsibilities. This need for an equivalent of parental power has been clearly described by a physician who experienced the same problems as a patient when faced with the uncertainty of treatment choice for his own cancer [17]: collecting a maximum of information and advice from many quarters resulted in a nearly intolerable indecision, which was only relieved when he accepted to rely on "a doctor", - " to seek a person who would dominate, who would tell him what to do, who would in a paternalistic manner assume responsibility for his care".

The same holds true for patients proposed for inclusion in a phase III randomised study: full information on the treatment choice and on the randomisation process means, in fact, recognition by physicians of their own uncertainty about the best treatment. In this case, all rational explanations on the scientific value of the randomisation procedure do not meet the patient's need for a paternalistic authority. Informed consent finally given could frequently mean that they rely on medical science as an equivalent of such an authority. Regression itself is a conflicting issue: patients rely on and like those people on whom they depend, but at the same time they may distrust or fear them, and hate their state of dependence.

Denial

Denial is frequently an intrinsic part of coping with cancer. Therefore, informed participation could be harmful for patients who cope with cancer by denial or by avoiding information [1]. This is especially true for some patients who do not know their diagnoses and are not keen to receive too many details or participate in treatment decisions.

In fact, denial is a complex device, and is more frequently selective than global, helping patients believe that they are in the subgroup destined to respond to therapy and to be cured [1]. Inability to adopt an objective view of the overall statistics concerning one's own fate is both a positive way of coping and an obstacle to adequate participation in treatment choices.

Secondary Gains of Cancer

Cancer can be considered as "a heavy-duty permission to avoid returning to a stressful job, and a legitimate reason for even the toughest person to ask for help and attention" [14]. In this sense, depending on others is a way of gaining or recovering some power over them. Such paradoxical capture of power at the same time when it is abandoned into the hands of friends, family or caregivers can lead to a tendency of sustaining disease and dependency, rather than returning to a world of helplessness and loneliness. Another patient has described cancer as a powerful problem-solver, since it may allow to satisfy emotional needs and to gain sympathy, love and attention, with the risk of subconsciously wishing to remain ill to retain attention [18].

Practical Problems in Increasing Patient Participation

Several practical problems may be encountered when one tries to increase patient participation:

- giving more information and responsibility to the patient may increase his/her anxiety, at least at the beginning [19]. It is a common experience that choices may be difficult especially when there are no guidelines and when the alternatives are of paramount importance for the decision-maker him/herself;
- patient participation is time-consuming: Time is necessary in the first place to avoid making decisions too quickly, with potentialisation of stress resulting from the first diagnosis of cancer. In addition, as we shall see later, eliciting the patients' preferences requires time for a better knowledge of their personalities and aims, and for a calm explanation of the various alternatives;
- finally, the behaviours necessary to maintain health, utilise health care facilities and comply with treatment plans are so numerous that the task of caring for oneself is frequently overwhelming [20]. Medical decision-making is a complex process, involving a large number of factors; it is difficult to rationalise for the physicians, and even more so for the patients.

Variables Affecting Patients' Information-Seeking and Treatment Choice

In addition to the ambivalence of each individual patient with respect to information and participation, there is a wide spectrum between those who do not want to know and delegate all decision-making and care to health providers and those who actively seek full information and want to participate in treatment choice. Several studies have been devoted to the analysis of variables which may account for such behavioural differences.

Age and Sex

Age is one of the most important variables. Among cancer patients, those who want all available information - good and bad - and prefer participating in decisions rather than leaving them to the doctor are significantly more numerous in the younger age groups [1]. It has also been observed that age is a major factor influencing eligibility and entry in clinical trials for cancer: patients aged 65 or older with an available protocol were less likely to be clinically eligible or placed in a study [21]. Such differences can probably be explained both by physicians' preferences and patients' refusal.

However, two - non-exclusive - hypotheses could limit the value of age being a factor *per se* for patient participation:

- On the one hand, it has been observed that age was not significantly associated with the patients' preferences, but correlated with the clinicians' estimates of such desire [15]. Thus, once again one should try to carefully distinguish a patient's true desire from what the clinician assumes it to be.
- On the other hand, different age-related behaviours could mainly illustrate a historical shift towards greater consumer participation. The younger patients could therefore mainly reflect the new sociocultural behaviour, rather than acting according to their age as an absolute factor.

Sex probably also interferes with information seeking: women are generally considered to engage in more extensive health search [22].

Educational and Socio-Economic Factors

It is a well known fact, confirmed by daily experience, that patients of the higher socio-economic classes, with higher incomes and superior educational levels, are more willing to obtain information and actively participate in decision-making [1,15,23]. In the study performed by Cassileth et al. on cancer patients, a better education appeared as the variable which correlated best with a preference for participating in treatment decisions [1]. Several explanations can be proposed for this, for example:

- greater ability to seek and to understand information, an attitude which strongly correlates with a desire to participate in decisions [1];
- greater congruence with the socio-economic status and beliefs of the health professionals [22];
- a mind socially oriented toward participation in commands and decisions.

Conversely, a lack of cultural and social resources such as observed in illiterate or foreign patients who do not speak the language of the medical institution, leads to adaptation problems and poor participation.

Ethnic Factors

Patients from the Third World are particularly confident in the medical possibilities of the developed countries. The cultural gap could lead to a risk of inability to get proper medical information and to participate in medical decision-making and treatment. However, a recent study performed in our department has allowed us to conclude that patients from Third World countries who were referred for treatment with high risks of morbidity and mortality, were better informed than expected [24]. There may be, however, less suspicion against possible medical errors among patients referred from the Third World than among patients from the developed countries. In the United States, some differences were also observed between white and non-white patients, the white race having higher education and income levels that correlate both with the patients' desire to help make decisions and with the clinicians' estimates of such desire [15].

Cultural Factors

Patient participation has been encouraged in our countries by consumerism. It has been emphasised that consumers can participate in their health care at different levels: the health care organisation or institution, the health care programme, and the individual health care provider [3]. There is, obviously, interaction between these different levels. For example, the feminist and consumer rights movements have been instrumental in raising women's expectations of participation in decision-making regarding treatment of a malignant breast lump [5]. The role of the mass media in disseminating health information and influencing health behaviour has been underlined, with newspapers, magazines and television being as important sources of information as the health care profession [5].

Personality Traits and Psychological Factors

Following a review of the literature on consumer behaviour, Lenz has identified several interrelated personality traits as the most likely to influence the extent of information-seeking behaviour [22].
Information seeking is:

- encouraged by tolerance for ambiguity, self-esteem, need for cognitive clarity;
- inhibited by rigidity, dogmatism, high level of anxiety, and/or alienation (external locus of control).

In cancer patients, several studies have tried to identify the personality traits and psychological factors which best correlate with active seeking of information and participation in medical decision-making and treatment. Using the Beck Hopelessness Scale, Cassileth et al. observed that cancer patients who wanted as much information as possible - good or bad - and who preferred active involvement in their own care were more hopeful than those who did not [1]. Although a better medical status was found to correlate with the level of hope, the correlation between the Hopelesness Score and desire of participation retained statistical significance when the medical status was kept constant.
The role of other psychological factors, such as anxiety, compulsive or overbearing personalities, as well as sociability can be also hypothesised.
Some studies have focused on psychological factors influencing women's primary options in breast cancer treatment. Preference for treatments that preserve the cosmetic appearance was found to be related to concern about body image [25] and self-interest, whereas women who elected mastectomy were more tense, anxious, introverted, felt more depressed and reported more sexual problems [26].

Interpersonal and Environmental Factors

Marital status, familial and social network may be expected to strongly influence patients' behaviour and preferences [22,27].
For example, privacy and comfortable family surroundings facilitate information exchange between client and health professional: these conditions are frequently lacking in hospitals and clinics [22]. In fact, a broader interpersonal environment has been shown to influence health-related search behaviour, while patients with few social contacts showed less tendency towards information seeking and participation.
In addition, the quality of the interpersonal environment may facilitate or impede information seeking [22] and participation. For example, a cooperative, supportive atmosphere encourages individuals to seek information from those in superordinate positions, possibly including health professionals.

Disease-Related Factors

One can expect less tendency towards patient participation in the attitudes of both patient and caregivers in the case of:

- poor prognosis (where there is some reluctance to give or ask for full information);
- no-choice situation, such as immediate initiation of standard treatment in the face of a threatening situation;
- acute disease or intensive treatment.

The recent trend to use intensive and high risk treatments such as bone marrow transplantation in some forms of cancer has made patient participation even more difficult, compliance being required in the face of a

Table 1. Factors interfering with patients' information and participation seeking

	VARIABLES INTERFERING	
	Positively	Negatively
1. **Background variables**		
- Age		Older
- Sex	Female	
- Education	Higher	
- Socioeconomic status	Higher	
- Ethnic Factors	Third world	
- Cultural Factors	Consumerism	
2. **Personality traits**		
- Attitude towards alternatives	Tolerance	Rigidity
- Cognitive style	Clarification	Dogmatism
- Self-perception	Self-esteem	
- Optimism/pessimism	Hopeful	
- Emotional disorders		Anxiety
- Locus of control	Internal	Alienation
3. **Environmental factors**		
- Family, social network	Extensive	
- Health-care setting	Supportive	
4. **Disease-related variables**		
- Interval since diagnosis	Short	
- Prognosis		Poor
- Course		Chronic
- Treatment choices	Consensus	No choice
- Physical condition	Better	

hopeless disease. Acute disease orientation has been already shown as opposed to a rehabilitative philosophy, patients in the acute wards being generally surrounded by overwhelming medical technology [28]. More generally, time constraints, the degree of uncertainty and risk involved in the decision, and the number of alternatives available might interfere with patient participation [22]. A longer time interval since the diagnosis could also be a source of less participation, the patient being progressively resigned and passive-minded. Conversely, in the study of Cassileth et al., patients who sought more detailed information were those who had their disease diagnosed more recently [1].

Modalities of Patient Participation

Seeking and Receiving Information

This is the first and frequently the main or single step of a patient's participation. According to Schain, the critical questions to be explored are the following [4]:

- What information will serve what purpose ?
- For whom is such information valuable and in what dose and context ?
- What is the appropriate time to introduce such information ?
- Whose responsibility is it ?
- How should such information be made available (oral, printed material, audio-tapes, etc.).

An inappropriate level of information can be due to several causes [29,30]:

- patient's passive attitude and lack of active search;
- forgetting or misunderstanding by the patient of the information provided;
- doctor's reluctance to share information for various reasons, e.g., fear of increasing the patient's anxiety, although frequently ignorance adds to stress [31], fear of revealing diagnostic and therapeutic uncertainties, inability to communicate across social and cultural barriers, and lack of time.

Conversely, patients frequently feel that the doctor is too busy to keep explaining things and choose to remain ignorant rather than "bother" the doctor [29]. Too frequently doctors presume that patients do not know because they do not wish to know [31].

As a result, lack of information may lead to increased anxiety, enhanced stress, maladjustment to treatment side effects , poor compliance [31], inadequate information drawn from alternative - uncontrolled - sources, and inadequate treatment choices.

It is also important to point out that the information indispensable to the patient concerns the possible side effects and the results expected from treatment, rather than the specific medical name of the treatment [1], or the pathophysiology of the disease. In fact, information on well known toxicities such as vomiting and alopecia is usually far better, although partial and sometimes biased, than information on other possible damage, e.g., renal, cardiac, neurological - which could explain the necessity for serial investigations [29].

Participation in the Initial Investigations

McNeil and Pauker have proposed a model which incorporates patients' attitudes in the evaluative process of diagnostic tests [32]. Thus, some patients with lung cancer are so averse to the risk of perioperative death that they should have preoperative testing to search for occult metastases, a search which, based on its indices of efficacy, should not be performed in the majority of cases with operable bronchogenic carcinoma.

Participation in the Medical Decision-Making Process

Participation in medical decision-making depends on the amount and types of information given to the patient [29]. A strong correlation has been observed in cancer patients between preference for maximum information and desire to participate in decisions [1]. However, another study performed on patients with hypertension has shown that, although a majority wanted to receive additional information about their illness and to discuss decisions about treatment, only a minority desired to participate in or make initial decisions [15]. Thus, clinicians might underestimate the patients' desire for information and discussion, but overestimate their desire to make decisions. In another study, patients expressed a need to participate in the decision-making process, but did not want to make the final decision about treatment [33].

A major factor impeding active participation of the patient in the initial medical decision-making is the stress frequently present at the time of diagnosis [34], especially in case of acute illness, e.g., acute leukaemia: a sense of urgency about the treatment decision creates enormous stress [5]. In less abrupt and in chronic situations, patient participation seems easier but will depend on individual personalities and degree of commitment. Participation groups have been proposed as a way of facilitating individual integration into the information/decision-making process. But even in general practice, such participation groups have stayed far behind what was initially expected, raising the question of whether they actually represented the desire of some physicians, health authorities and organisations rather than the needs of the patients [34]. However, these problems and limitations should not lead to the conclusion that patient participation is a pipe dream [35]. There has been historical modification of the situation in recent decades, with most patients nowadays getting full information on their diagnosis, prognosis and treatment choices [36].

Participation During Treatment

Compliance with the therapeutic regimen is a major factor of effectiveness, and the ratio of received to planned total dose of chemotherapy (dose intensity and number of courses) has been correlated with response and duration of response. Yet it has been argued that some doctors are attracted to patient participation in order to increase the patients' compliance, i.e., to gain power over them [9]. Hayes-Bautista has described different modalities of noncompliance as attempts of the patient to gain some control over treatment [13]. In most cases of anticancer treatment these tactics, whether demands, disclosures or suggestions, are related to actual or feared side effects, and may result in bargaining, the outcome of which will depend on the range of treatment choices and the trade-off capacities of the physician. For example, an oncologist can accept a delay of 1 or 2 weeks of a fourth or consecutive course of chemotherapy, if a complete remission has been achieved, and if this supplementary time is needed by the patient for vacation which will improve his/her quality of life and guarantee the ensuing completion of treatment.
Hence, it can be seen that patient participation during treatment is usually restricted to good compliance, which frequently means personal psychosocial adaptation to therapeutic strain and full development of coping strategies. There is, at the moment, little active participation required, although:
- relaxation and positive visualisation have been proposed as a way of directly involving the patient in the treatment course, at least through a decrease of side effects [34];
- involvement of the patients, through self-controlled blood counts, in monitoring chemotherapy; induced myelosuppression has been advocated as a safe way to alleviate the staff burden and improve the patients' self-esteem and control [19];
- participation of patients is frequently required for self-care, such as monitoring and cleaning a central venous access;
- continuous infusion of cytotoxic drugs through portable pumps is a new therapeutic modality which could increase patient participation;
- self-modulation of the infusion rate of opioids through a portable pump has been proposed as a good method of achieving optimal pain control.

Rehabilitation

Rehabilitation is a major therapeutic step in the recovery from cancer. It must be undertaken during the treatment programme and after its completion. In fact, as already emphasised, even participation of the patient at the time of the first treatment choice may aid recovery [37].
Rehabilitation can be analysed at different levels:
- somatic (e.g., choice of a wig following chemotherapy-induced alopecia or of a breast prosthesis following mastectomy, voice recuperation following laryngectomy, self-care for stomy, adaptation to a limb amputation etc.);
- family (e.g., adaptation to sexual disturbances following treatment of pelvic cancer, child adoption following disease- or treatment-related sterility, and any family adjustment in spite of permanent impairment);
- professional (e.g., ability to return to work, to accept reduced activity or to look for a different job better suited to the new situation);
- social (e.g., ability to accept financial strains in relation to the disease, the treatment or the new situation, reorientation of leisure activities, etc.).

Active participation is needed for each of these levels and is a condition for the full success of rehabilitation.

Patient Participation During the Terminal Phase of the Disease

Resignation would seem more advisable to the patient than active participation during the late or terminal phase of the disease. Yet important choices are commonly made at this stage, such as discontinuing chemotherapy or electing a phase I or II clinical trial, starting an analgesic treatment with morphine, staying at home or entering a palliative care unit in a hospital or hospice.

It has been suggested that all treatment decisions concerning seriously ill and dying patients should be based on their own wishes or best interests, rather than on an external judgment as to their quality of life [38]. Reaching a high quality of communication is therefore necessary to allow these patients to express their preferences. Based on a patient's aknowledgement of the progression of the disease and the imminence of death, informed choice between the use of experimental drugs and no further chemotherapy has been proposed even to children with cancer [39]. In fact, such choices are frequently difficult to prescribe during the terminal phase, and it has been proposed to determine patient preferences far in advance [38]. This is especially needed when one foresees final incompetence. Taking into account the frequent incompetence of terminal cancer patients - whether due to delirium, to acute complications, or to debilitation or depression, should one rely on their previously expressed preferences such as the "Living Will"? What should the patient's involvement be in the "Do-Not-Resuscitate Order"? In fact, probably due to the reluctance of caregivers to discuss these decisions with patients, competent patients are often bypassed in the Do-Not-Resuscitate Orders, when such a policy is unofficially adopted [40]. Requests for euthanasia or assisted suicide are even more difficult to deal with, most of these wishes being expressions of suffering and subrogate demands for help, and raise a number of ethical and legal issues [38].

Accompanying patients during the last phase of their disease and trying to determine with them their ultimate goals in life are the right ways to approach these problems. The patients' participation in the analysis and evaluation of their pain represents an important part of their involvement in treatment choices. The role of the family is also particularly important at this stage. The major decisions are frequently made through concertation of caregivers (physicians, nurses, psychologists, social workers) and family, following close communication and disclosure of the patients' desires. In that sense, patients' despair can be viewed as a failure of their environment to elicit their preferences and to communicate with them.

Patient Participation In Clinical Research

Patient participation in clinical trials is relatively low. Recent surveys on the demography of patients enrolled in the NCI-sponsored clinical trials have shown that only a minority who were eligible for protocols actually entered these studies [21]. Defining eligibility criteria in a restrictive way for legitimate scientific reasons probably reduces the diffusibility of these studies. As a result, it has been questioned whether patients under study are representative of the entire cancer population [41]. Clinical trials are more frequently performed in cancer centers and University hospitals, and patient participation in these studies could be related to socio-demographic variables - age in particular - [21] and to active seeking on the part of the patients which leads them to be treated preferably in these institutions.

Informed consent is an ethical and legal requirement before entering a patient into a clinical trial. Similar to compliance with treatment in general, it does not truly represent active participation, since patients are only allowed to accept or refuse a protocol which has been planned by physicians on a scientific basis. However, one wonders whether entering clinical trials does not correspond to an attitude of active participation in scientific progress. This is especially true for patients entering a phase I trial, the aim of which is merely determination of drug pharmacology and toxicity: such entry is based on voluntarism and a kind of altruism. In phase III studies, the preferences of some patients may be overridden by the random allocation to one of the treatment arms [26], and such preferences are seldom properly questioned: the final decision could be based on a subjective rather than objective, scientific basis, and patient accrual could be reduced. The same holds true for participation in a study randomising a treatment regimen versus observation: although no statistical difference was observed for anxiety levels for patients enrolled in such trials comparing adjuvant chemotherapy in early breast cancer with observation [42], some individual patients may have preferred one modality to the other. Properly sought informed consent is the best way to approach these issues, but one must be aware that enrolling patients into clinical trials implies requiring their active participation in a scientific study as well as in their own treatment.

Patient Participation in Early Detection of Cancer Disease - or Relapse

Early detection is one of the best prognostic factors for such cancers as breast, cervix, colo-rectal or melanoma. Informing the general public through the media, as well as adequate training of general practitioners are commonly recommended in order to reach the optimum level of early detection.

Breast self-examination has been proposed as one of the best ways to improve early detection, but its effectiveness has been questioned. Comparisons between women who express interest and adopt a free breast self-examination teaching programme and those who do not, have shown that the former are characterised by more family history of cancer, a longer relationship with their physicians, more confidence in the effectiveness of cancer detection and treatment, and more personal responsibility for health outcomes [43]. These data provide some support for the cost-effectiveness of self-selection for such teaching programmes. When a breast lump has been detected, the woman can be involved in the decision-making process through a two-step procedure in which a period of several days elapses between the biopsy and surgical removal of the malignancy and/or breast [5]. In this case, ambulatory biopsy might be the best procedure for decreasing both anxiety and economic cost [44].

Methods have also been compared for participation in screening programmes for colo-rectal cancers through search of faecal occult blood or sigmoidoscopic examination, the most effective being the use of an information-invitation letter sent by the patient's family doctor with return postage included for the reply [5]. Such studies provide a basis for improving participation in early detection programmes, by delivery of information via the general practitioner, and reinforce the hypothesis that the best participation is obtained through an optimal patient-caregiver interaction, with a selective role devoted to the general practitioner.

The same holds true for early detection of relapse. This is usually obtained through good compliance of patients with the follow-up programme in the clinics where the primary cancer has been initially treated . However, the role of the patient and of the general practitioner in such follow ups has not been carefully investigated to date. Regular investigations in specialised clinics can cause unnecessary anxiety or provide reassurance, depending on the patient's personality, and may contribute to impeding his/her rehabilitation. The cost-effectiveness of the various types of follow-up has not yet been assessed.

Patient Participation in Children, Adolescents, Elderly and Incompetent Patients

Partitipation of Children and Adolescents

Two specific aspects concerning the participation of children with cancer in their treatment have been underlined [46]: firstly, children are physically, economically and legally dependent on their parents; when a life-threatening disease occurs, the entire decision of how to manage this disease remains within the adult world. Secondly, most children with cancer are treated according to research protocols within clinical trials, whereas only a minority of adults with cancer enter such trials. Research normally implies voluntary participation and freedom to refuse continuation at any time. For children, informed consent is legally required from their parents, with frequent trade-offs between the parents, the caregivers and the sick child.

The possible solutions to the psychological and ethical problems raised by this situation can be found in a better perception of the child's attitude in the face of a serious disease: contrary to the traditional assumption, children should be considered more like adults in their feelings, and less like adults in their thoughts - which implies that factual information should be given in simplified, age-appropriate language [46]. Children will therefore participate in medical decision-making just as adults do, on the basis of their emotional projections and confidence in their loved ones, with the only legal restriction that

caregivers will seek their assent, the formal consent being given by their parents.
Adolescents differ from both children and adults [20]: they are at the stage where one tries out his/her own capacity for autonomy and self-competence, while the limitations of their responsibility are questioned by themselves and by others. According to Jordan and Kelfer, "their developmental capabilities and limitations, their enthusiasm for independence, and their fragile egos all contribute to their somewhat confusing self-care potential... Rejection of authority and self-assertion are the tools for coping with the loss of childhood and subsequent search for identity." This background must be taken into account when one is faced with the frequent non-compliance with anticancer treatment in adolescents, and/or with rejection of parental authority. Caregivers frequently have to bargain for the best medical decision and especially for compliance with the treatment protocol. Establishing and preserving good communication offers the best chances of both completing the therapeutic programme and achieving an optimum state of development in spite of the disease and the therapy. Adolescents as well as children exemplify that the key problem is integration of disease-related experiences into a developmental process rather than rehabilitation as a theoretical return to a pre-disease state.
Finally, both young children and adolescents are able - often better than their parents and caregivers would expect - to adapt to the worst situations, including treatment failure and imminence of death [39]. However, the chemo and radiosensitivity of most cancers occurring at that age, the relatively good tolerance to highly toxic regimens, as well as the refusal by adults to accept a fatal outcome, lead with increasing frequency to repeated attempts of intensive and potentially curative treatments such as bone marrow transplantation. Risk acceptance of such treatments raises important ethical issues, usually in an intensive emotional context. Staff meetings involving physicians, nurses and psychologists, good communication with the patients, concertation with their families are prerequisites for reaching the right medical decision with patient participation.

Participation of elderly patients

Elderly patients most often also have reduced autonomy, due to decrease of their physical - and also socio-economical - capabilities. Yet, contrary to the younger patients, they have longer experience with the vicissitudes of life and fully developed value judgments [38]. Their participation in crucial decisions such as starting a risky procedure for a poor prognosis disease or discontinuing therapy is a daily ethical problem in oncology, in view of the frequency of cancer in this age group. Frequently, caregivers are reluctant to give full information which could increase patient anxiety, and rely on their own value judgments for the important medical decisions. The family is commonly involved in this decision-making process. A patient's values can be ascertained through dialogue about his/her goals, wishes and expectations from probable outcomes of treatments, and risk acceptance - frequently reduced in elderly patients [47].
Caregivers can also rely on the values reported by the family, and, whenever they have been expressed, advance directives such as a "Living Will". However, direct involvement of the patient in each therapeutic step through mutual communication and participation should be preferred as far as possible to medical decision-making formally based on advance directives and surrogates.

Incompetent patients

The ethical issues are even more difficult when the patients become incompetent. In this case, a surrogate - usually a family member - makes decisions for them. These decisions should be based on substituted judgement, i.e., on what preferences the patients had in the past, now applied to the matter at hand [38]. Unfortunately, such preferences have seldom been clearly expressed. Even in these cases, they should not relieve the caregivers from the ethical obligation of defining the best option. Local ethical committees could provide some help in case of a difficult choice, but concertation of caregivers and family members is the main way of achieving an agreement on the best solution, based on what is known of patient's values and preferences, and on objective assessment of the medical situation.

Improvement of Patient Participation

Is Patient Participation Needed ?

This preliminary question has been partially answered in the first section of this chapter devoted to the potential benefits of participation. Yet the best judges of the interest or necessity of patient participation are the patients themselves. The opinions recently published by patients who belong, or are close to, the medical profession are diverse: some strongly recommended to help the patient fight his/her cancer through appropriate means of participation [14]. Even in the case of incurable disease, it was held important that the patient take charge of the situation, in order to improve as much as possible both his/her quality and quantity of life [18]. But others have experienced and emphasised that some degree of authoritarianism, paternalism and domination is essential to good medical care [17].
In fact, these statements must not be viewed as contradictory: ambivalence, already mentioned, explained that each individual needs, to varying degrees, some autonomy and some authoritarianism.
However, whatever the compromise needed by each individual patient, one must be aware that contemporary medical practice may become discordant with lay expectations [6], and that nobody can substitute for the patient in defining his/her own utility. This last point has been clearly shown in a study performed by Ciampi et al., in which fictitious patients were assigned a low utility because of social isolation, physical handicap and lack of motivation, and were therefore considered as appropriate targets for a radical, high-risk treatment, a conclusion obviously unacceptable from an ethical viewpoint [27]. Another study has shown that the vast majority of patients feel that they have an important part to play in the treatment of their illness [29]. There is no doubt, therefore, that patient participation is needed, at least for a better identification of his/her wishes and expectations.

How to Inform Patients about their Disease and the Treatment Choices ?

As already emphasised, patient participation starts with information. However, one must be careful about the possible cultural gap between the medical approach and the patient's view of his/her illness [6]. In addition, individuals are frequently overwhelmed by the amount of new information, which could surpass what they can assimilate, especially in the context of anxiety at the time of diagnosis [5]. Objective statistical data on the probability of outcomes and risks must be integrated in the individual's hopes and fears, and the assimilation of risk acceptance to a plain gamble [47] is questionable.
Therefore, information must always be integrated in the general context of physician-patient communication and interaction: communication includes but goes beyond objective information and represents the first step in the therapeutic relationship. Communication is established by words, attitudes, expressions and gestures: it demands effort, thought and time [4]. Simultaneously with the establishment of good communication which is the basis of the patients' confidence in the possibility of expressing their thoughts, questions and wishes, written information helps to provide them with a set of objective information that they can examine at their own pace and discuss with family members and nurses. In addition, it is recommended that physicians write in the patients' records a summary of what has been told, and give them a copy of standardised information that is orally delivered (Schain). It is important to ask patients what they do know and want to know [15], in order to give them an appropriate presentation of diagnosis, treatment and side effects [14].

Psychological Preparation

Psychological preparation is a simultaneous process and represents an early component of physician-patient interaction. The use of guidelines for pivotal discussion concerning diagnosis and treatment plan was shown to help patients with testicular cancer and their spouses to manage the stress of treatment, and attain a better degree of satisfaction with

interpersonal relationships despite sexual and reproductive limitations [10].
Such preparation must include an analysis of the patient's personality traits, and identification of psychosocial factors which may interfere with medical decision-making. The drawing of a family-tree and the evaluation of professional position and economical strains are recommended during this phase; the use of a series of psychosocial assessment tools can be also helpful [26].
Psychological preparation is a task for all the caregivers, not only the main physician, i.e., the oncologist, in charge of the patient: the role of the general practitioner, nurses and other members of the hospital staff is also very important. Associations of cured patients, such as Reach-to-Recovery, are very helpful for such preparation, and their contacts with the patients must be facilitated. Finally, patients should be able to identify at least one person to whom they can talk and ask advice, in addition to obtaining medical information [29].

Elicitation of Patient Preferences

Elicitation of patients' preferences could be viewed in a simplistic way: just ask the patient what his/her wishes and expectations are, following the necessary information about diagnosis and prognosis. This will help to reduce discrepancies between his/her views and those of the physician, since these discrepancies may cause problems for clinical management [6]. Frequently, this elicitation can be better achieved by involving other caregivers besides the oncologist primarily in charge, especially the nurses and the general practitioner, and by discussion with the closest family members. Psychologists and social workers can be of great help during this phase. The use of self-report inventories can be warranted, in order to measure the patient's expectations and the degree of responsibility and participation he/she assumes for personal health care [26], but such scales cannot replace direct contacts and interviews. The same applies to the patients' attitudes towards risk(s) [27], but simple questions about preference in theoretical situations can be rejected by the patients as purely artificial in the context of the real situation they are faced with.
The way information is presented to patients may strongly influence their preferences: in a study by McNeil et al., where 2 treatments - surgery or radiotherapy - were proposed for lung cancer, with a higher immediate risk but better average 5-year survival rate for surgery, more patients preferred radiotherapy when treatments were not identified and when the outcomes were presented in terms of the probability of dying rather than the probability of living [48].

Involving Patients in the Medical Decision-Making Process

Medical decision-making means choosing between different alternatives, including sometimes a no-treatment arm. This decision, either intuitive or formally based on a decision-tree, will be made more or less easily depending on whether the therapeutic index (advantage/disavantage ratio) of the "best" treatment prevails markedly or slightly over the value of alternative treatments. The "utility" (value) of the outcome of each treatment is based on current medical knowledge of the expected results (survival, risk of relapse) and costs (side-effects and financial costs). Whenever the relative utility of a new - experimental - treatment, compared to a standard treatment, preferably based on a wide consensus, is totally uncertain, patients should be encouraged to enter a prospective randomised trial. In any case, the utilities of the various alternatives must integrate the value judgment and preferences of the individual patient. Yet, one must avoid the illusion that the patients themselves, following full information, will make the medical decision: with few exceptions, the best treatment choice must be selected by the physician and offered to the patient. It should be selected on the basis of consensus developed through clinical trials and consensus conferences. When a microscope examination is necessary, it should preferably be performed through fine needle aspiration cytology or Trucut needle biopsy, in order to give the patient the opportunity to know the results and to discuss the treatment options. This 2-step procedure has been recommended especially in breast cancer, in order to save women from having mastectomy without previous discussion [49]. Once the discussion is started, the question raised is how, in practical terms, the patient's preferences can be integrated in the medical decision-making process, in order to result in individually tailored utilities.

Several methods have been proposed to incorporate such preferences. Trade-offs between quantity and quality of life have been investigated, by asking patients with stage T3 carcinoma of the larynx to express their preferences for various lengths of survival with normal or artificial speech [50], such analysis indicating that to maintain their voices, 20% of them would choose radiation instead of surgery. Risk acceptance can be evaluated when 2 therapeutic modalities, e.g., surgery and radiotherapy, are compared in terms of immediate risk of death and long-term chances of survival [47]. Outcome values can be expressed as "objective" units, such as mortality rates, disability days, 5-year survival and costs, or as "subjective" units corresponding to the patient's own value judgment on his/her quality of life [51]. The assessment of subjective individual values is especially important when equal survival probabilities for the 2 options are assumed. Corder and Ellwein have incorporated individual patient utilities for the potential toxicities of the various investigation and treatment modalities for Hodgkin's disease, and have shown that such weightings result in different choices between MOPP chemotherapy without staging laparotomy, and staging laparatomy followed by radiotherapy when appropriate [52]. Four categories of potential toxicity for the 2 treatments were very differently weighted from one individual to another: cutaneous toxicity, hair loss, pulmonary and reproductive toxicity, whereas other important toxicities such as infections or neurological effects may not influence the decision.

However, these methods have so far been utilised for studies in fictitious patients, and their applicability to real patients is questionable. Furthermore, the options are based on the known (past) toxicities of present treatments, which are currently challenged by treatment modalities with less toxicity and a better therapeutic index. For example, in the case of Hodgkin's disease, individual choice of MOPP chemotherapy without staging laparotomy is questionable if one takes into account the constant sterility and the 2-5 % risk of secondary leukaemia resulting from such treatment, even if these toxicities are weakly weighted in some individual patients. Therefore, the development of new therapeutic strategies appeared more advisable to the community of oncologists, and the current EORTC protocol proposes, without staging laparotomy, a stratification according to prognostic factors, with treatment arms combining in most cases radiotherapy and a chemotherapy regimen devoid of reproductive toxicity and far less leukaemogenic than MOPP.

In addition, subjective involvement of the patient in medical decision-making is a dynamic process, within the general framework of coping with the situation and establishing a patient-caregiver therapeutic relationship: adaptation to foreseen toxicities (e.g., hair loss, vomiting, etc.) must be made by both the patient and the caregivers who may propose several preventive or supportive possibilities.

Adjuvant Methods for Patient Participation in their Health Care

Patient participation must not be restricted to primary medical decision-making and compliance with the planned treatment. Cancer patients should be encouraged to gain control over their own bodies and to cope with the psychosocial disorders induced by their disease or the treatment. Relaxation, biofeedback or autogenic training, and healthy imagining can be proposed as adjuvant methods, at least in some individuals who could benefit from them [14], but these methods should not substitute for objective information, primary curative or palliative treatment, and a good patient-caregiver therapeutic relationship.

Role of the Family

The family plays an important role in the information and decision-making process. Frequently, and especially in case of cancer and poor prognostic diseases, family members receive more information than the patients themselves; such situations most probably correspond to a desire of both caregivers

and family members to protect the patient from unbearable reality. Yet excess in such imbalanced information is ethically questionable and can lead to a total loss of patients' responsibility.
In fact, in each individual case, an analysis of family roles is necessary in order to identify the common values, the most important relatives and the eventual conflicts. Patients should be made aware of the complex interaction between caregivers, family members and themselves. They should be offered, even implicitly, the possibility of restricting some or all information to those selected persons whom they will designate. Participation in the medical decision-making should be restricted to themselves, or shared with the most significant relatives in accordance with their habits and wishes.
The involvement of the family is especially important in the case of patients with decreased level of responsibility, i.e., children, elderly and incompetent patients. The spouse's role is also prominent in such cancers as breast, gynaecological or testicular, where treatment choices can deeply interfere with marital/sexual relationships. Psychological preparation of the relatives as well as the patients is crucial, for it will contribute significantly to the patient's and family's ability to adapt to the diagnosis, to manage the stress of treatment, and to attain a greater degree of satisfaction following cure [10]. For example, most sexual partners want to be involved in the decision-making leading to mastectomy [5].

Role of Self-Care Groups and Associations

Self-care groups may be considered as another - indirect - way of patient participation. They provide a more formal basis for the frequent exchange of information and support between patients.
Some groups or movements are especially directed towards particular varieties of cancer, e.g., Reach-to-Recovery for breast cancer, associations of laryngectomised people for head and neck cancers etc. These provide newly diagnosed patients with an efficient support based on experience of cured patients, who, by their own example, stimulate coping and participation. Patients do learn from each other and the hospital staff ought to exploit this opportunity [28].
Groups of relatives have also proved useful, for example, parent groups in childhood malignancies, or combined parent/adolescent groups [20].
Following a patient's death, mourning groups are currently proposed to the closest family members (parents or spouses) and may constitute a helpful and efficient way for family members to shorten the duration of grief and reduce the potential pathological consequences.
Finally, patient participation groups represent a way of incorporating the layman in the medical decision-making process, whether for an individual patient, or for collective choices through integration with professionals in consensus conferences [49]. They may also influence health policy, through assessement of the quality of services and of patient satisfaction, and provide equipment and support to improve care and help medical research. Groups for patient participation in general practice have been developed especially in Great Britain as a way of promoting health, and have even resulted in a National Association for Patient Participation [53]. The interest and impact of such groups is still a matter of debate: whether their active members - frequently doctors rather than patients - represent the views of others (the "incompetent periphery") and meet the needs of patients, whether they can influence the behaviour of caregivers and the decisions of physicians and other decision-makers, are still open questions [53]. However, in general practice as well as in oncology, these groups represent a positive reality in 5 main areas: consumer feedback, health promotion, community care, providing information and fundraising.

Conclusion

Encouraging patients to seek information and participate in treatment choices meets a public demand today. Patients, and especially cancer patients, need a comprehensive therapy corresponding to a holistic approach of medicine [14]. As oncologists become increasingly specialised, such comprehensive therapy is provided by multidisciplinary teams and implies patient participation. Several patient-physician models do exist, e.g., authoritarianism, compliance, participation and self-help. Participation, viewed as a contractual relationship where both the physician and the patient face their responsibilities, corresponds altogether to the most operational and most ethical one.

REFERENCES

1 Cassileth BR, Zupkis RV, Sutton-Smith K and March V: Information and participation preferences among cancer patients. Ann Int Med 1980 (92):832-836

2 Zittoun R: L'information des malades en hématologie. Bordeaux Med 1982 (15):51-57

3 Brody DS: The patient's role in clinical decision-making. Ann Int Med 1980 (93):718-722

4 Schain WS: Patient's rights in decision making : the case for personalism versus paternalism in health care. Cancer 1980 (46):1035-1041

5 Valanis BG and Rumpler CH: Helping women to choose breast cancer treatment alternatives. Cancer Nursing 1985 (8):167-175

6 Kleinman A, Eisenberg L and Good B: Culture, illness, and care. Clinical lessons from anthropologic and cross-cultural research. Ann Int Med 1978 (88):251-258

7 Schulman BA: Active patient orientation and outcomes in hypertensive treatment. Med Care 1979 (17):267-280

8 Stuart-Harris R, Simes RJ, Coates AS, Raghavan D, Devine R and Tattersall MH: Patient treatment preference in advanced breast cancer: A randomized cross-over study of doxorubicin and mitozantrone. Eur J Cancer Clin Oncol 1987 (23):557-561

9 Clayton S: Patient participation: an underdeveloped concept. J Royal Soc Health 1988 (108):55-56

10 Cassileth BR and Steinfeld AD: Psychological preparation of the patient and family. Cancer 1987 (60):547-552

11 Morris J and Royle GT: Offering patients a choice of surgery for early breast cancer: a reduction in anxiety and depression in patients and their husbands. Soc Sci & Med 1988 (26):583-585

12 Price JLW: The patient's morale. Lancet 1977 (1):533

13 Hayes-Bautista DE: Modifying the treatment: patient compliance, patient control and medical care. Soc Sci & Med 1976 (10):233-238

14 Fiore N: Fighting cancer - one patient's perspective. N Engl J Med 1979 (300):284-289

15 Strull WM, Lo B, and Charles G: Do patients want to participate in medical decision making ? JAMA 1984 (252):2990-2994

16 Laplanche J, Pontalis JB: Vocabulaire de la Psychanalyse. Presses Universitaires de France Ed Paris 1984

17 Ingelfinger FJ: Arrogance. N Engl J Med 1980 (303):1507-1511

18 Skinner B: How to participate in your own health: a cancer patient's view. Lancet 1984 (2):971-972

19 Harder L and Hatfield A: Patient participation in monitoring myelosuppression from chemotherapy. Oncol Nurs Forum 1982 (9):35-37

20 Jordan D and Kelfer LS: Adolescent potential for participation in health care: Issues Compr Pediatric Nurs 1983 (6):147-156

21 Hunter CP, Frelick RW, Feldman AR, Bavier AR, Dunlap WH, Ford L, Henson D, Maccfarlane D, Smart CR and Yancik R: Selection factors in clinical trials: results from the Community Clinical Oncology Program Physician's Patient Log. Cancer Treat Rep 1987 (71):559-565

22 Lenz ER: Information seeking: a component of client decisions and health behavior. Adv Nurs Sci 1984 (7):59-72

23 Green LW: How physicians can improve patients' participation and maintenance in self-care. West J Med 1987 (147):346-349

24 Ruszniewski M, Mambou G, Cordier R, Lepee B, Filliou M, Zittoun R: Study on informed consent process of patients referred from third world countries to a French haematological department. Second Scientific Meeting Eur Soc Psychosoc Oncol Amsterdam, Oct 1988

25 Margolis GJ and Godman RL: Psychological factors in women choosing radiation therapy for breast cancer. Psychosomatics 1984 (25):464-469

26 Wolberg WH, Tanner MA, Romsaas EP, Trump DL and Malec JF: Factors influencing options in primary breast cancer treatment. J Clin Oncol 1987 (5):68-74

27 Ciampi A, Silberfeld M and Till JE: Measurement of individual preferences. The importance of "Situation-specific" variables. Med Decision Making 1982 (2):483-495

28 Davis MZ: The organizational, interactional and care-oriented conditions for patient participation in continuity of care: a framework for staff intervention. Soc Sci Med 1980 (14 A):39-47

29 Karani D and Wiltshow E: How well informed? Cancer Nurs 1986 (9):238-242

30 Robinson EJ and Whitfield MJ: Improving the efficiency of patients' comprehension monitoring: a way of increasing patients' participation in general practice consultations. Soc Sci Med 1985 (8):915-919

31 Cancer Research Campaign Working Party in Breast Conservation: Informed consent: ethical, legal, and medical implications for doctors and patients who participate in randomised clinical trials. Br Med J 1983 (286):1117-1121

32 McNeil BJ and Pauker SG: The patient's role in assessing the value of diagnostic tests. Radiology 1979 (132):605-610

33 Vertinsky IB, Thompson WA and Uyens D: Measuring consumer desire for participation in clinical decision-making. Health Serv Res 1974 (9):121-134

34 Poletti R: L'influence des facteurs émotionnels et du stress dans la maladie cancéreuse. Krankenpflege 1979 (72):435-440
35 Patient participation: more pipe dream than practice? Br Med J 1981 (282):1413
36 Novack DH, Plumer R, Smith RL, Ochitill H, Morrow GR, Bennett JM: Changes in physicians' attitudes toward telling the cancer patient. JAMA 1979 (241):897-900
37 Hames A, Stirling E: Choice aids recovery. Nursing times 1987 (83):49-51
38 Thomasma DC: Ethical and legal issues in the care of the elderly cancer patient. Clin Geriatric Med 1987 (3):541-547
39 Nitschke R, Humphrey GB, Sexauer CL, Catron B, Wunder S and Jay S: Therapeutic choices made by patients with end-stage cancer. J Ped 1982 (101):471-476
40 Evans AL and Brody BA: The Do-Not-Resuscitate Order in teaching hospitals. JAMA 1985 (253):2236-2239
41 Friedman MA: Patient accrual to clinical trials. Cancer Treat Reports 1987 (71):557-558
42 Cassileth BR, Knuiman MW, Abeloff MD, Falkson G, Ezdinli EZ and Mehta CR: Anxiety levels in patients randomized to adjuvant therapy versus observation for early breast cancer. J Clin Oncol 1986 (4):972-974
43 Grady KE, Kegeles SS, Lund AK, Wolk CH and Farber NJ: Who volunteers for a breast self-examination program? Evaluating the bases for self-selection. Health Educ Quart 1983 (10):79-94
44 Stein HD: Ambulatory breast biopsies: the patient's choice. Am Surgeon 1982 (48):221-224
45 Madlon-Kay DJ: Methods to encourage screening sigmoidoscopy examination. J Clin Gastroenterol 1986 (8):701-702
46 Van Eys J: Ethical and medicolegal issues in pediatric oncology. Hemat/Oncol Clin North Amer 1987 (1):841-848
47 McNeil BJ, Weischelbaum R and Pauker SG: Fallacy of the five year survival in lung cancer. N Engl J Med 1978 (299):1397-1401
48 McNeil BJ, Pauker SG, Sox HC Jr, Tversky A: On the elicitation of preferences for alternative therapies. N Engl J Med 1982 (306):1259-1262
49 Consensus development conference. Treatment of primary breast cancer. Br Med J 1986 (293):946-947
50 McNeil BJ, Weischelbaum R and Pauker SG: Speech and survival: Tradeoffs between quality and quantity of life in laryngeal cancer. N Engl J Med 1981 (305):982-987
51 Speedling EJ and Rose DN: Building an effective doctor-patient relationship: from patient satisfaction to patient participation. Soc Sci Med 1985 (21):115-120
52 Corder MP and Ellwein LB: A decision-analysis methodology for consideration of morbidity factors in clinical decision-making. Am J Clin Oncol (CCT) 1984 (6):19-32
53 Richardson A and Bray C: Promoting health through participation. Policy Studies Institute. London 1987, Research Report N° 659

Patient Information: Practical Guidelines

C. Hürny

Medical Department C.L. Lory, Inselspital Bern, Freiburgstrasse, 3010 Bern, Switzerland

In every medical textbook the clinical interview, history taking and clinical examination are described as the most essential basis of medicine. In contrast to these statements, little time is devoted to the training of clinical skills in medical education. Interviewing a patient is still considered as an art, and physicians as being gifted or not. In our experience, interviewing skills can be taught and learned.

Since information of the patient with cancer is a biopsychosocial problem, we use a comprehensive interview technique that enables the physician to assess the biomedical, psychological and social situation at once in the first encounter with the patient [1,2]. The difficult steps of the interview are listed in Table 1. In step 1, the physician greets the patient, introduces himself and defines his professional role. This may seem a matter of simple politeness in human interactions. However, observations in a busy clinic show that these rules are not always followed. In step 2, the physician explores how the patient is feeling at that particular moment and he puts the patient at ease. An optimal interview situation is important to enable the patient to give his

Table 1. Interviewing techniques [1,2]

Step 1	The physician	- greets the patient - introduces himself - defines his professional role	
Step 2		- explores how the patient is feeling - makes the patient feel comfortable	
Step 3		- invites the patient to mention all symptoms of his present illness	
Step 4		- examines the present illness in detail - listens to the patient's spontaneous references to concurrent life circumstances, illnesses in the past and issues of family health and relationships (Past Health, Family Health, Personal and Social History)	
Step 5		- inquires in detail about	Past Health
Step 6			Family Health
Step 7			Personal Development
Step 8			Social History
Step 9			System Review
Step 10		- asks whether the patient has questions, or anything to add - informs the patient about the next steps	

subjective view of the disease. The interview technique is open-ended, i.e., the physician must follow the patient's associations. This makes registration of data more difficult, but gives the physician a unique opportunity to assess the subjective experience of the disease in the biographical context of the patient. In step 3, the physician asks the patient to mention all symptoms of the present illness. In step 4, he examines the present illness in detail. He listens to the patient's *spontaneous* references to concurrent life circumstances, illness in the past, issues of family health and relationships (Past Health, Family Health, Personal and Social History). In steps 5-9, the physician inquires in detail about Past Health, Family Health, Personal Development, Social History and System Review. Usually, after steps 1-4, the steps are not followed in chronological order. If possible, the physician follows the patient's spontaneous report. Before concluding the interview the physician asks whether the patient has questions, or anything to add, and finally informs the patient of the next steps.

In this first clinical interview, the basis is established for subsequent information of patient and family about the nature of the disease.

Once the diagnosis of a specific cancer in a specific stage is made, how does the physician proceed to the actual information? In Table 2, some practical guidelines are listed. These are derived from our personal experience and the subjective experience of Sanes, a physician who has gone through the process of having cancer [3].

Appropriate timing to avoid unnecessary interruptions is of utmost importance. A matter of such importance cannot be dealt with on casual occasions such as daily rounds. If the patient agrees, the spouse, partner, or significant others may be included to avoid so-called "double bookkeeping". Often the spouse asks the doctor not to tell the patient, because he believes that the patient is not able to cope. Conversely, the patient may ask the physician not to inform the spouse for the same reason. These demands are often due to projective defences. The patient projects his own difficulty to be confronted with the diagnoses onto his spouse and *vice versa*. If the physician colludes with these demands, a state of non-communication, detrimental to both partners, is maintained. Both "know", but believe that the other does not. Open communication is a prerequisite for coping with an acute crisis. A first step in the approach of telling the diagnosis to the patient and his family is to inquire about the patient's own thoughts about the disease, with the following wording: "It has been some time now that you are ill, what do you think you have?" The possibility of cancer has occurred to most patients before the physician makes it explicit. In our opinion, the word "cancer" should be used and clarified for the specific, actual situation. Otherwise the irrational phantasies and symbolic meanings of cancer will persist in an undetermined way, fostering uncertainty. It is important to meet the patient at his own level of understanding; medical terms should be avoided or explained. Finally, disclosure of the

Table 2. Discussing the cancer diagnosis with the patient: guidelines [3]

1. APPROPRIATE TIMING (avoid unnecessary interruptions)
2. PRESENCE OF PARTNER/SPOUSE
3. PATIENT'S OWN THOUGHTS ABOUT HIS DISEASE
4. USE OF THE WORD "CANCER"
   EXPLANATION OF THE SPECIFIC SITUATION (pencil and paper may be helpful)
5. USE OF SIMPLE WORDS (avoid or explain medical terms)
6. LISTEN TO QUESTIONS OF PATIENT AND FAMILY (e.g., regarding alternative treatments)
7. AVAILABILITY OF CAREGIVERS (physician, nurse) FOR QUESTIONS OF PATIENTS AND FAMILY OVER TIME

diagnosis is only the beginning of a long information process. Patient and family will have questions throughout the course of the disease until cure and sometimes thereafter, or until death. The availability of caregivers over time is crucial. "Being informed" is not a steady state of the patient. It varies substantially depending on the circumstances, and may range from absolute denial to total awareness.
Since the treatment of cancer is multidisciplinary in most cases, the communication between the various specialists involved and the family physician is of great importance, but is often neglected. Not only are biomedical data to be transmitted, but also psychosocial issues, i.e., the actual state of information of the patient. Sanes, a physician with malignant lymphoma, gives an impressive report of his subjective experience as a patient with hospitals, medical specialists and general practitioners [3]. According to him, the patient is able to cope with the fact that the physician cannot cure him. But he cannot cope if the caregivers do not look after him.

REFERENCES

1 Morgan WL, Engel GL: The Clinical Approach to the Patient. WB Saunders, Philadelphia 1969
2 Adler RH, Hemmeler W: Theorie und Praxis der Anamnese. Der bio-psycho-soziale Zugang zur Krankheit. Fischer Verlag, Stuttgart 1986
3 Sanes S: A Physician Faces Cancer in Himself. State University of New York Press, Albany 1979

Diagnosis and Management of Symptoms from a Psychological Perspective

Jimmie C. Holland

Psychiatry Service, Memorial Sloan-Kettering Cancer Center, 1275 York Avenue, New York, NY 10021, USA

This review of symptoms that represent psychological distress is written in such a way that clinicians can recognise and apply the interventions. It also covers the situations in which it would be helpful to ask for psychiatric consultation. The first thing to keep in mind is that you are generally dealing with psychologically healthy individuals who are facing a serious or even catastrophic event. For these individuals, you, as the physician responsible for their care and treatment, are in the best position to offer the information about illness, treatment and expectations. When conveyed with a sense of concern and compassion, this will be sufficient to support most patients psychologically through the crises of illness. It is good to remember, however, that even the most courageous and strong individuals in the face of unremitting pain may show severe signs of psychological distress. These resilient individuals can be identified by their history of facing previous life crises and illnesses with a mature and direct response. Other individuals, also readily apparent by history and manner of coping poorly, can be expected to tolerate even mild levels of discomfort and stress with difficulty. They need to be recognised early and earmarked for early support and intervention, which may prevent problems later. Since patients who are coping better, alone or assisted, are more apt to comply with their medical treatment and participate well in their care, it behooves the oncologist to pay attention to this aspect of patient care, since it impacts not only on the quality of the patient's life while being treated, but also contributes to the outcome of treatment itself. This chapter, and the ones by Maguire on distress and recognition of it, attempt to equip the clinician to use the present knowledge in this area of his practice.

First, it is important to know the normal responses, in order to be able to identify the abnormal ones (see also the chapter by Bolund on adaptive and maladaptive coping). The response to a crisis in cancer, either at the time of diagnosis or at some later crisis point, has a typical pattern: initial disbelief and denial, warding off the bad news transiently, followed by emotional turmoil characterised by anxiety, fears, a sense of hopelessness, insomnia, anorexia and even transient weight loss. This is usually dissipated by recognition of the beginning of a treatment plan and by the awareness that something can be done. Adaptation goes on over the ensuing months and the degree to which it is positive depends on prior personality, support from the doctor and family, and control of distressing treatment side effects [1]. A short-acting benzodiazepine, such as lorazepam and alprazolam, in low dose for daytime, or a hypnotic at bedtime for insomnia is helpful.

Abnormal Responses

Reactive Anxiety and Depression

On the borderline between normal and abnormal reactions are the most common emotional disturbances in cancer patients: reactive anxiety and depression, which exceed what we assume to be normal. In the United States these are called adjustment disorders with depressed and/or anxious mood. These symptoms are an exaggeration of the emotions seen in the normal stress response, but greater in intensity or duration. Symptoms are usually depressive in nature, with a depressed mood, hopelessness and guilt. They may be accompanied by anxiety that varies from mild to severe. In the study of prevalence of psychiatric disorders among cancer patients, about half the patients had sufficient distress to meet the criteria for a psychiatric disorder, using the US standard classification [2]. Of that half with distress, two-thirds had reactive anxiety and depression. Treatment is short-term supportive psychotherapy in which emotional support, clarification of the medical facts and mobilisation of the person's own coping abilities are provided. Often, involving the patient's family members also enhances support. If the distress is great enough to impair daily function, a psychotropic drug may be added, either a short-acting benzodiazepine or an antidepressant such as amitriptyline which also improves sleep. Cognitive and behavioural interventions can be useful because patients are highly motivated to help themselves by using relaxation exercises and by intellectually viewing the crises in a more constructive way.

Depression

While it is normal to be sad because of illness and the losses associated, true depression is far more rare and the clinician should be able to recognise the difference; the latter should be treated aggressively, especially since suicidal risk or abandonment of treatment may be the consequences. Similar to the data about pain and greater distress, our data pointed out that the 20-25% who have symptoms of major depression fell predominantly among those with greater disability, advanced disease and pain. The prevalence of depression was similar to the incidence in equally ill patients with other diseases [3]. That study also showed that the physical symptoms of depression which are used in healthy individuals to identify depression, i.e., anorexia, weight loss, fatigue and loss of interest and libido, are not useful in cancer patients because they are also symptoms associated with most cancers. The diagnosis of depression in cancer patients must be made on the basis of the psychological symptoms: dysphoric mood, hopelessness, worthlessness, guilt and suicidal ideation. In such patients, one must take a careful history to assess possible aetiology: drugs such as corticosteroids, vincristine or vinblastine, asparaginase, intrathecal methotrexate, interferon. Also, metabolic encephalopathy and paraneoplastic syndromes can present by altered mood. Patients vulnerable to developing depression are also those who have pancreatic cancer. Holland and coworkers [4] in the Cancer and Leukaemia Group B found that patients with pancreatic cancer, compared with gastric cancer patients who were similar on all medical variables, were more distressed and depressed, confirming the long-suspected association of a possible biologically-related depression as a paraneoplastic syndrome with pancreatic tumours. In addition, vulnerable patients are those who have had previous depressions or a family history.

Patients with depression should be treated with a combination of supportive psychotherapy, enhancing social supports around the individual and antidepressant medication (Table 1). The tricyclic antidepressants are most frequently used, starting at a low dose at bedtime and increasing by 10-25 mg every 1 to 2 days until benefit is seen. Depressed cancer patients often reach therapeutic response levels at very low doses. Patients are maintained on the drug for several months, then it is lowered and discontinued. Amitriptyline and doxepin are useful for sedating effects, while patients with psychomotor retardation will benefit from those with least sedating properties, protriptyline and desipramine. Drugs with low anticholinergic side effects in patients with gastrointestinal symptoms are desipramine and nortriptyline. Second-generation antidepressants are appropriate if the tricyclics are unsuccessful. MAOIs should be continued in patients previously taking them, but diet may restrict their use in patients with previous dietary problems. Lithium carbonate must be continued in patients receiving it previously. It can be continued to the time of surgery and restarted when oral medication can be given. It should be used with caution with nephrotoxic chemotherapeutic drugs. It has not proved clinically useful in neutropenic patients, pro-

Table 1. Medications used in cancer patients

Generic name	Starting daily dosage (po)	Therapeutic daily dosage (po)
Tricyclic antidepressants		
Amitriptyline	25 mg	75-150 mg
Doxepin	50 mg	75-150 mg
Imipramine	25 mg	75-150 mg
Desipramine	25 mg	75-150 mg
Nortriptyline	50 mg	100-150 mg
Second-generation antidepressants		
Trazodone	50 mg tid	150-250 mg
Maprotiline	25 mg qd	50-75 mg
Amoxapine	25 mg tid	100-150 mg
Bupropion	100 mg tid	300-450 mg
Monoamine oxidase inhibitors		
Isocarboxazid	10 mg bid	20-40 mg
Phenelzine	15 mg bid	30-60 mg
Tranylcypromine	10 mg bid	20-40 mg
Lithium carbonate	300 mg bid	600-1200 mg
Sympathomimetic stimulants		
Dextroamphetamine	2.5 mg bid in the morning	
Methylphenidate	5 mg bid in the morning	
Benzodiazepine		
Alprazolam	0.25-1.00 mg tid	0.75-6.00 mg
Fluoxetine	20-49 mg qd	20-40 mg

Reprinted with permission from Breitbart and Holland, 1988 [5]

viding only transient response. Psychostimulants have a place in withdrawn patients with advanced disease. Dextroamphetamine often potentiates the effect of narcotic analgesics and counters the sedating effect of narcotics as well.

The benzodiazepine alprazolam has been useful for anxiety and depression. Mianserin is a drug of considerable value in depressed cancer patients [6]. In addition, fluoxetine appears of considerable value as well in cancer patients, though experience is limited.

One of the exciting new uses for antidepressants has been the control of pain, both as an adjunct to narcotic analgesics and as a primary treatment for peripheral neuropathy of chemotherapeutic origin and postherpetic pain. The action has been shown to be independent of its antidepressant effects [7].

Anxiety

Anxiety occurs in many different forms in cancer. It is heightened by the cultural view of it as a dreaded disease. Presently, there is also a great interest in mind-body connections and cancer, which lead people to fear that the stresses in their lives cause cancer. Anxiety appears first and by far most in cancer in relation to the crises of illness: at the time of diagnosis, relapse and treatment failure, as discussed earlier, usually mixed with depression (see above).

Anxiety also occurs related to medical factors: poorly controlled pain is critically important to consider in any patient who is distressed. Abnormal metabolic states that produce anxiety are hypoxia, pulmonary embolism, sepsis, delirium, hypoglycaemia, bleeding and heart failure.

There are also several tumours which secrete hormones and, acting as paraneoplastic syndromes, produce anxiety: pheochromocytoma, thyroid tumours, parathyroid adenoma, ACTH-producing tumours and insulinoma.

History must be taken to rule out an anxiety-producing drug: corticosteroids; neuroleptics used as antiemetics, producing akathesia; thyroxine; bronchodilators; beta-adrenergic stimulants; paratecal reaction to antihistamines; and withdrawal states from alcohol and drugs.

Another situation associated with anxiety is the paradoxical increase in anxiety on completion of a lengthy treatment regimen. Patients respond with anxiety on recognition of loss of the protective treatment and close monitoring by the staff [8]. Some patients find the Magnetic Resonance Imaging (MRI) and CT scan frightening, especially those with a history of claustrophobia. About 20% of patients have significant trouble in tolerating the procedures [9].

Preexisting anxiety disorders are often exacerbated by cancer and its treatment, such as needle phobia, agoraphobia, panic disorder, generalised anxiety disorder, hypochondria and posttraumatic stress disorder.

Treatment is of three types; psychotherapy; behavioural techniques; and psychopharmacology. Often they are combined for best effect. Psychotherapy is largely supportive, providing information, rehearsal of feared events and reassurance. It is usually targeted to the crisis period. Behavioural methods are used in relaxation exercises, hypnosis and systematic desensitisation. All are helpful in reducing anxiety, enhancing a sense of self control and cognitively reframing the patient.

There are several helpful drugs: most widely used are benzodiazepines. The addition of short-acting forms of lorazepam, alprazolam and oxazepam has been useful. Also of help for anxiety control are beta-blockers, tricyclic antidepressants, monoamine oxidase inhibitors, antihistamines and neuroleptics.

Delirium (Organic Mental Disorder)

Often overlooked as a subtle cause of psychological symptoms is altered central nervous system function caused either by direct invasion of cancer, or by its indirect effects through a metabolic encephalopathy, occurring as a complication of the cancer or treatment. Posner, of the Neurology Department at Memorial Sloan-Kettering, estimates that 15-20% of hospitalised cancer patients have some degree of cognitive dysfunction, most of which is unrecognised. Of the consultations reviewed in over 500 patients by the psychiatric group, 20% of the requests were for evaluation or management of confusional states. A consultation requested for mood change often reveals early mental confusion. It is important to think of this cause of mental changes because the underlying aetiology is often treatable. It is, of course, first necessary to rule out alcoholic delirium tremens or drug withdrawal, by careful history.

The causes of delirium are several. In relative order of frequency in cancer patients, they are most commonly related to medication. Narcotic analgesics are the worst offenders, especially in high dose (levorphanol, morphine, meperidine). These are followed by steroids in high or tapering dose. Acute psychotic symptoms, often with fearful hallucinations of imminent harm, are common. Next in frequency is electrolyte imbalance, followed by failure of a vital organ or system, particularly renal or pulmonary. Acute infections with septicemia cause confusional states, as do poor nutritional states, cardiovascular complications of cancer and paraneoplastic syndromes from hormone-producing tumours. In a study by Massie and coworkers [10], it was found that delirium occurs with a frequency of more than 75% in terminally ill patients. It also was found, as we have experienced in clinical practice, that the aetiology is most likely to be not one but a combination of factors. For example, in this study, analgesics, infection, hypoxia and haemorrhage were present in combinations that made it impossible to establish a clear cause.

Symptoms of delirium in early stages can be recognised by a sudden change in mood or behaviour, either becoming withdrawn or agitated. Suspiciousness and uncooperativeness in a previously pleasant individual should be noted. The first assumption is often depression or emotional distress, but early mental changes may be the cause. This may progress to florid agitation and psychosis, which are difficult to manage on a medical floor. Early treatment is highly desirable and may need to begin while the workup is in progress. One-on-one nursing observation is the first order to assure no violent behaviour or leaving the ward. Psychotic and agitated patients require a short but rapidly acting drug which can be safely administered. Haloperidol in low dose, with lorazepam to add sedation, is now our regimen of choice, though circumstances may alter this choice. It can be given orally, by injection or by intravenous route with safety if given slowly and with careful monitoring, beginning with 0.5 mg in a very debilitated person to 5 mg in a large, acutely disturbed individual. Movement disorders can be prevented by use of diphenydramine and trihexyphenidyl. Akathesia responds to low doses of propranolol 10-20 mg t.i.d., diazepam or benztropine. The neuroleptic malignant syndrome rarely occurs at the low and briefly sustained dose.

Nausea and Vomiting

The improved control of posttreatment nausea and vomiting associated with several chemotherapy agents and combinations has been one of the major contributions to the quality of life of patients receiving chemotherapy. The increasingly sophisticated antiemetic regimens have employed phenothiazine, benzodiazepine and steroids in combination. Behavioural interventions have been useful adjuncts. Metochlopromide has been widely adapted to this use in large dose, which over several cycles can result in acute dystonias and akathesias which will go unrecognised as functional anxiety if not considered as a common cause of posttreatment agitation and unusual movements.

Patients receiving chemotherapy regimens with particularly high emetogenic potential, such as cisplatin, adriamycin and bleomycin, were noted early on to develop anticipatory nausea and vomiting. Behavioural psychologists undertook study of this phenomenon and found it to be a classical Pavlovian conditioned response occurring in between 15 and 65% of patients, depending on the drug with which they were being treated. Since it was sufficiently severe in some patients to cause them to stop treatment, behavioural methods were employed and found quite successful. Irrespective of the specific behavioural technique employed (e.g., progressive relaxation and visual imagery or systematic desensitisation), patients improved and could control these distressing symptoms of becoming nauseated and even vomiting on route to the hospital. Several factors increase the risk of getting it: high anxiety, high expectation, prior problems with food sensitivities and motion sickness. Redd and colleagues [11] also found that posttreatment nausea and vomiting, recognised to vary even when patients receive identical dose and identical antiemetic control, is responsive to the same vulnerability factors.

The depth of this response is remarkable. In a study of Hodgkin's disease survivors as long as 12 years later, Cella and colleagues [12] found that these healthy survivors still reported anxiety and nausea when an inadvertent smell (such as the nurse's perfume or the cleaning solutions used in the clinic) or sight (the appearance of the nurse or doctor who gave the treatment or the sight of the street to the clinic) reminded them of treatment.

Pain

In the prevalence study of PSYCOG [2], those patients who had sufficient distress to warrant a psychiatric diagnosis (half of the group under study) were examined for presence of pain. When the patients with psychiatric diagnoses were examined separately, 39% had pain rated above 50 on a 100 mm line, as opposed to only 19% of those without psychiatric diagnosis, indicating the fact that presence of pain alters the psychological state. These data confirm our clinical observation that the psychiatric symptoms of patients who are in pain must initially be considered as a consequence of uncontrolled pain. Acute anxiety, depression with despair (especially when the patient believes the pain means progression of disease), agitation, irritability, uncooperativeness, anger and insomnia are all symptoms of pain. These symptoms in a patient with pain should not be labelled as a psychiatric disorder unless they persist after the pain is controlled. The patient's mental state can only be assessed accurately after the pain has been controlled.

Table 2. Cancer pain

Psychotropic adjuvant analgesic drugs			
Generic name	Trade name	Approximate daily dosage range (mg)	Route
Tricyclic antidepressants			
Amitriptyline	Elavil	10-100	po, im, pr
Imipramine	Tofranil	12.5-100	po, im
Doxepin	Sinequan	12.5-100	po, im
Trazodone	Desyrel	25-200	po
Phenothiazines			
Fluphenazine	Prolixin	1-3	po, im
Methotrimeprazine	Levoprome	10-20 q6h	im,iv
Butyrophenones			
Haloperidol	Haldol	1-3	po, im, iv
Antihistamines			
Hydroxyzine	Vistaril	50 q6-4h	po, im, iv
Psychostimulants			
Methylphenidate	Ritalin	2.5-10	po
Dextroamphetamine	Dexedrine	2.5-10	po
Steroids			
Dexamethasone	Decadron	4-16	po, iv
Methylprednisolone	Solu Medrol	16 mg BID	po
		40-80 mg daily	iv
Amine precursors			
L-Tryptophan		500-3,000	po
Benzodiazepines			
Alprazolam	Xanax	0.25-2.0 mg t.i.d.	po

Reprinted with permission from Breitbart and Holland, 1988 [5]

While pain is the major fear of all patients, its frequency is not as great as believed. Patients with early disease have pain in about 15% of cases, while it increases to 60% in metastatic disease, and this may become difficult to manage in a much smaller percentage during terminal illness. It is important that all disciplines working in cancer understand the principles of pain management. Optimal management requires attention of the pharmacological, psychological, behavioural and anaethesiological approaches and rehabilitation to effect control. While a full review is not given here, psychotropic drugs, particularly the antidepressants, are useful. Table 2 gives the psychotropic drugs and their use in pain. As noted, they have independent analgesic properties, but the group also is effective for control of associated anxiety, depression, insomnia and delirium. The tricyclic antidepressants (imipramine, amitriptyline, doxepin and trazodone) are potent serotonergic agents, and also affect a number of neurotransmitters which mediate their analgesic effect. Phenothiazines such as methotrimeprazine are equianalgesic with morphine, have none of the opiate effects on gut motility, and probably produce analgesia through alpha-adrenergic blockade [5]. Used only with caution, they can produce hypotension and sedation. Dexamethasone and methylprednisolone also provide a sense of well-being and improved appetite. Hydroxyzine is a mild anxiolytic with sedating and analgesic properties that is useful in the anxious patient with pain. Alprazolam is a helpful adjuvant to control phantom limb or deafferentiation pain.

Sexual Problems

Cancer patients are often embarrassed to ask questions about their sexual problems, feeling that they are frivolous in comparison to their treatment of cancer. Physicians and their staff are often also embarrassed to ask about problems because they were never trained in how to ask questions about sexuality. The result is a frequent standoff between the patient who does not ask and the doctor who also does not ask [13]. The problems patients are experiencing are of two kinds: gonadal dysfunction with infertility related to surgery, radiation, or chemotherapy, or damage to sexual organs or function; and psychosexual problems which stem from fears, misinformation, or a feeling of sexual inadequacy related to change in appearance or perception of adequacy. These issues indeed do not surface during the immediate crisis of life and death and treatment decisions and early rehabilitation. However, they begin to become important when the patient perceives that the crisis is resolved and normal everyday responsibilities and activities are expected. It is then that the concerns about sexuality may begin to be more acute, and also when the astute oncologist should ask about it. Questions about fertility and sexual function are particularly relevant to the young patients who have been treated for testicular cancer, Hodgkin's disease, leukaemia treated by whole-body radiation, and those with pelvic tumours that may have altered sexual organs or their function. They are also particularly relevant to single patients who must face the issues of forming new relationships, low self-esteem, altered appearance and dating new individuals. Of concern are the great number of women who have been treated for breast cancer and who, by virtue of altered appearance of breasts, often have difficulty in resuming or initiating sexual relations because of the problems of self-esteem resulting from breast surgery or radiation [14].

Auchincloss, using the methods of Kaplan, suggests that it is important to be able to take a sexual history which elicits the chief complaint, the medical, psychological and sexual status, as well as present relationships and past sexual function. Knowing that information, she recommends that the patient, with the partner, be engaged in the discussion and that a positive stance be taken, since most sexual problems related to cancer can be managed, recognising that sexual expression is always possible and anxiety impedes a normal sexual response. She recommends taking a good sexual history which is comprised of obtaining information about the three parts of a sexual response: level of desire (often altered in cancer patients as a response to fears); excitement; and orgasm. Often simple explanations or recommendations are sufficient, but if they are not adequate, be sure that a colleague with training in human sexuality and who knows the common problems of cancer is available for referral of more complicated cases.

Insomnia

The inability to sleep is a common problem in cancer patients. It may relate to anxiety about illness, treatment, or the future. It may also have other causes, such as medication (steroids, interferon, AZT), and a careful drug history is helpful. Patients may be afraid to fall asleep because they equate it with death which is an ever-present fear. They may fear nightmares about the future or their concerns. Whatever the cause, it is important to identify the particular concerns and discuss them. It is also important to determine whether the insomnia relates to trouble going to sleep (like anxiety) or middle or early awakening (more likely depression). A careful history to elicit drug reaction, anxiety and depression as causes should clarify aetiology. Reassurance, coupled with a hypnotic or an antidepressant with sedative properties, should be adequate for control. Triazolam, flurazepam, or amitriptyline or doxepin at bedtime should encourage sleep. The effect upon ability to cope is recognisable and daytime cheerfulness and adequate coping may result from this minimal intervention. Cancer patients often fear the addicting qualities of these drugs when in point of fact, like with analgesics, they must be encouraged to continue them long enough for effect. Addiction is not a problem in these psychologically healthy individuals.

Fatigue

Fatigue and loss of stamina are symptoms which are understandable in the patient undergoing active treatment. They are more difficult to understand in the survivor, yet they are common and persistent complaints. Discussion is found in a later section on survivors.

Summary

In conclusion, a number of symptoms plague the patient with cancer and interfere with his or her quality of life. Importantly, they may also interfere with treatment compliance. It behooves the treating oncologists to be familiar with the symptoms of anxiety, depression, delirium, sexual problems, insomnia and fatigue, to both recognise them and offer helpful interventions or referral to experts who can treat these troublesome and ofttimes demoralising symptoms.

REFERENCES

1 Massie MJ and Holland JC: Psychiatric complications and their management. In: Holland JC and Rowland JH (eds) Handbook of Psychooncology. Psychological Care of the Patient with Cancer. Oxford University Press, New York 1989

2 Derogatis LR, Morrow GR, Fetting J et al: The prevalence of psychiatric disorders among cancer patients. JAMA 1983 (249):751-757

3 Bukberg J, Penman D and Holland JC: Depression in hospitalized cancer patients. Psychosom Med 1984 (46):199-212

4 Holland JC, Hughes-Korzun A, Iross S et al: Comparative psychological disturbance in pancreatic and gastric cancer. Am J Psychiatry 1986 (143):982-986

5 Breitbart W and Holland JC: Psychiatric complications of cancer. Curr Ther Hematol Oncol 1988:268-275

6 Romero J, National Cancer Institute, Mexico City, Mexico. Personal communication

7 France RD: The future of antidepressants: Treatment of pain. Psychopathol 1987 (20 Suppl 1):99-113

8 Holland JC: Psychological aspects of cancer. In: Holland JF and Frei E (eds) Cancer Medicine, 2nd ed. Lea & Febiger, Philadelphia 1982 pp 1175;2325

9 Redd NH: Behavioral approaches to treatment-related distress. Ca - A Journal for Clinicians 1988 (38):138-145

10 Massie MJ, Holland JC and Glass E: Delirium in terminally ill patients. Am J Psychiatry 1983 (140):1048-1050

11 Redd WH and Andrykowski MA: Behavioral intervention in cancer treatment: Controlling aversion reactions to chemotherapy. J Consult Clin Psychol 1982 (43):595-600

12 Cella DF, Pratt A and Holland JC: Persistent anticipatory nausea, vomiting, and anxiety in cured Hodgkin's disease patients after completion of chemotherapy. Amer J Psychiatry 1986 (143):641-643

13 Auchincloss S: Sexual dysfunction in cancer patients: Recognition and management. In: Holland JC and Rowland JH (eds) Handbook of Psychooncology. Psychological Care of the Patient with Cancer. Oxford University Press, New York 1989

14 Gates C: The "Most Significant Other" in the care of the breast cancer patient. Ca - A Journal for Clinicians 1988 (38):146-153

Employing Specialist Workers to Detect Psychological and Social Morbidity

Peter Maguire

Cancer Research Campaign, Psychological Medicine Group, Christie Hospital, Manchester M20 9BX, United Kingdom

Despite a growing awareness of the prevalence of psychological and social morbidity among patients with cancer, much of this morbidity remains unrecognised and untreated. Thus, in a prospective study of 75 women undergoing mastectomy, none of those who developed sexual problems were recognised as having done so by anyone involved in their care [1]. Similarly, in a further study only 15% of women who developed anxiety, depression, body-image or sexual problems during routine hospital follow up after mastectomy, were recognised and referred for help [2]. A recent prospective follow-up study of 120 patients with cancer of the cervix revealed that only 21% of patients had fully disclosed their concerns by the end of the first year after diagnosis [3]. If recognition of psychological and social morbidity is to be improved, the reasons for the failure to detect it need to be identified and understood.

Reasons for Hidden Morbidity

Both patients and health professionals contribute to this problem.

Patient-Led Barriers

Patients and relatives believe that the psychological and social problems that develop are an inevitable consequence of the cancer and associated treatments. So there is no point in mentioning them, since nothing can be done. Doctors and nurses usually begin consultations by focussing on a history of the cancer and whether or not there are signs of recurrence or physical complications of treatment. This leads patients and relatives to believe that it is not legitimate to raise non-physical concerns. Many doctors and nurses are busy and patients do not wish to overburden them because they are genuinely concerned about their welfare. They also fear that time spent on psychological and social problems might mean less time is spent on ensuring their physical survival. For all these reasons they tend to keep their concerns hidden.

Professional-Led Barriers

In-depth discussions with doctors and nurses [4] and direct observations of doctor-patient, nurse-patient and social worker-patient consultations [5] have found two major barriers, the avoidance of direct questions and use of distancing tactics. Thus, it is rare for a patient who has presented with a probable cancer to be asked questions like "What did you think it was?" or "How did you feel when you found it?"

If a patient or relative tries to raise a concern by giving a verbal ("I keep worrying about it coming back") or non-verbal cue (looks anxious of tearful), the health professional uses strategies designed to keep these concerns at a safe emotional distance.

Common distancing tactics include:

Premature Reassurance

Instead of acknowledging and clarifying the concern ("In what way do you keep worrying about it coming back"), the health professional insists "There's no need to worry, you are going to be alright." The professional does this because the prognosis is good and he is not aware that the patient had two close friends who were similarly reassured but died soon after. This response does not reassure the patient and blocks dialogue.

Normalisation

Here, the obvious distress of a patient or relative is explained away by the health professional as an inevitable and normal response in those circumstances.

Patient	I'm worried about radiotherapy.
Doctor	Every one is at first but you will be alright.

But this patient became even more fearful about radiotherapy. She had read that radiation was a cause of cancer and believed radiotherapy would make her disease progress.

False Reassurances

When health professionals realise that the outcome of the disease or treatment is poor, they may be tempted to deny the reality of their patient's predicament by using false reassurances.

Patient	(newly admitted to hospice) I am sure I have only come here to die.
Doctor	Don't be so gloomy. I'm sure you'll get well enough to go home again

If the nurse had responded by asking "Why do you think that?", a proper dialogue would have developed. It would have become clear that the patient was aware of how imminent her death was and was reconciled to it.

False reassurance is also offered when serious complications are less likely, as in this example.

Patient	(a businessman) I am very worried that my bag will smell and that I'll have an accident.
Stoma nurse	Oh, there's no need to worry. We have such good bags and perfumes these days.

This patient subsequently had problems with smell and became very distrusting of the nurse. Had she acknowledged ("So, you're worried that your bag will smell and about having an accident") and legitimised his concerns ("Yes, there could be problems"), she would then have offered appropriate reassurance ("That's exactly why I am here, I want to help you to avoid such problems but if they do occur we can try to find a solution.").

Selective Attention

Patients and relatives often offer cues about physical and non-physical concerns together. There is then a high risk that cues about non-physical concerns will be ignored.

Surgeon	How have you been since your surgery?
Patient	My wound seems to have healed well and radiotherapy went alright. But my arm is still swollen and painful and I've been feeling a bit out of sorts.
Surgeon	Tell me more about the problems you are having with your arm.

The surgeon proceeded to elicit a good history about the physical morbidity but never returned to "I've been feeling out of sorts". Had he asked "In what way out of sorts", he would have found she had become very depressed and was suffering from a depressive illness.

Premature Advice

Nurses in particular are prone to move into "advice mode" the moment a patient voices concerns, because they believe that the provision of information will resolve them.

Patient	(awaiting mastectomy) I'm worried about the operation.
Mastectomy nurse	There's no need to be. Let me tell you what will happen when you go into hospital ...

This patient had profound concerns about how her body image would be affected but was given no opportunity to raise these. She remained very worried despite all the information given, little of which she registered or remembered. She subsequently felt devastated by her breast loss.

Switching

When suddenly faced with an obvious and distressing concern, the health professional may switch the topic to safer ground.

Physician	How are you today?
Patient	I am still feeling utterly exhausted. My breathing is not any better. In fact I don't think I am progressing at all. I'm beginning to think I'm not going to make it. Am I going to make it?
Physician	Tell me more about this problem with your breathing.

Yet, this man realised he was not going to recover from his lung cancer. He simply wanted reassurance that as much as was possible would be done to prevent him from suffocating and suffering undue pain. In another example, the social worker responded to disclosure of a body image problem by switching to a new and safer topic.

Patient	(after mastectomy) I know they removed all the cancer but I cannot get used to how I look. I feel so repulsive.
Social worker	Have you talked to your family about your illness?

Jollying Along

When health professionals sense that a patient or relative is feeling anxious or gloomy they tend to react intuitively by advising "Come on, there's no need to be so gloomy, let's see a smile. Come on now."
This reinforces beliefs that it is not legitimate to disclose concerns and that "a brave face" must be maintained at all costs.

Reasons for Avoidance

Those doctors, nurses and social workers who participated in in-depth interviews and/or observation of their consultations with patients were all committed to improving psychological and social aspects of care. So, their distancing could not be attributed to ignorance or a lack of concern. Instead, it seemed related to their concern for their patients and deficiencies in their training.
They feared that asking direct questions about psychological and social aspects would take up too much time. It might upset patients and cause them to worry about issues which they would not have considered. It could prompt patients to ask difficult questions like "Is it cancer?", "How long have I got?" or "Why didn't you diagnose it sooner?" Such questions are difficult to answer, particularly if you do not know how best to respond to them. Directive questions like "How are you feeling?" may permit patients to express strong feelings of anger or despair. The problem is then how to help a patient work through such feelings without taking too much time and provoking a loss of emotional control and even greater distress.
Responding to and clarifying cues about distress would bring the health professional in close touch with the true nature and extent of a patient's or his/her relatives' problems. How should they then handle these, especially if there is no one to whom they can refer patients or relatives who have problems? There is a risk that getting close to the real consequences of cancer and its treatment might be upsetting and cause the health professionals to question the value of treatment, their own worth and personal philosophy, as the following quotations exemplify.

Medical oncologist	I know this treatment (cisplatinum) causes havoc but what am I to do? It is their only chance of survival. There is little I can do to reduce toxicity. If I keep finding out from my patients how awful it is I may feel I can no longergive it. Then where would they and I be?
Surgeon	I still believe that surgical removal of the breast for lumps over a certain size offers the best chance of cure. I also know that it can devas-

tate some women psychologically. At least they will be alive. If I establish how devastated they are I may find I cannot do the operation any more. So, it is better for me to stick to the surgical aspects, isn't it?

Hospice nurse: Of course most of my patients die. But so long as I do my best to ensure they die without undue physical suffering, I feel it is worthwhile. Now psychological suffering is another matter. I see it as inevitable and see no point in going into it. Besides, it might end up by my becoming desperate that I can do so little about it. It might make me give up this kind of work.

Physician: What is the point of finding out that patients are depressed if there is no one to refer them to?

Specialist nurse: Why probe below the surface if there is nothing that I can do about the problems I find?

Such enquiry makes it clear that health professionals feel that their training has not equipped them with key interviewing, assessment and counselling skills or taught them how to deal with difficult situations like: being asked difficult questions; being confronted with anger, despair, withdrawal or denial; breaking bad news; or dealing with collusion where a health professional or relative requests that the patient should not be told the diagnosis or prognosis. So, it is not surprising that they avoid direct questions and use distancing tactics. Moreover, few doctors, nurses and social workers have easy access to clinical psychologists or psychiatrists. Nor do they find they receive much support from colleagues for this psychological and social role. Indeed, they may be criticised for spending too much time talking with patients and not enough time "doing something useful".

Solutions

Three possible ways of increasing recognition have been or are being investigated. They include the appointment and training of specialist nurses and social workers, the training of other health professionals involved in cancer care and the use of self-rating questionnaires. This chapter focusses on the first solution. The others are discussed elsewhere in this monograph.

Specialist Nurses

The appointment and training of specialist nurses or social workers to monitor the progress of patients with cancer and their relatives and refer those who need help is an attractive solution. For, if doctors, nurses and social workers involved in cancer care are not prepared to get involved in psychological aspects, the specialist nurse or social worker can provide a link between these professionals and the patient and ensure that problems are recognised and fed back to the doctor, be it the hospital specialist or general practitioner. Such specialist workers will only be effective if they are properly trained.

Training

This must cover both the required knowledge and skills.

Knowledge

If specialist nurses and social workers are to be effective in their monitoring role, they must be aware of and understand:

1. The key psychological hurdles which patients with cancer and their relatives have to overcome if they are to adapt to the disease. These include uncertainty about outcome, a search for meaning, how to contribute to survival, stigma, how open to be about diagnosis and treatment, how to relate to close relatives and friends, and the availability and use of both lay and medical support.
2. The nature and prevalence of psychological and social morbidity associated with cancers and their treatments.
3. The signs and symptoms which distinguish morbid reactions requiring intervention from normal reactions which require no intervention.

4. The kinds of intervention which may be required and the indications for their use.
5. The areas which should be covered routinely when assessing how a patient is adapting. These include: a history of the patient's illness and treatment to date; patient's perceptions, psychological reactions and view of the future; and the impact of illness and treatment on the patient's daily life, mood and key relationships.
6. Barriers to disclosure and the reasons for these, including the distancing tactics commonly employed.

Skills

1. Certain skills are essential for effective interviewing and assessment and include: how to acknowledge, organise and clarify verbal and non-verbal cues given by the patient; how to encourage patients to be precise so that they recount the key events accurately and connect with and disclose the associated feelings; keeping patients and relatives to the point without alienating them so that optimal use is made of the time available; and how to encourage the expression of feelings.
2. Specialist nurses and social workers also need to learn how to open and close consultations so that a patient is aware of what is wanted and how much time is available if needed.
3. They must be able to ensure that both professional and patient agendas are covered. Thus, an effective specialist nurse will encourage a patient to disclose all his concerns first and will then clarify their nature and extent before ensuring that her own professional agenda is covered, be it related, for example, to chemotherapy, pain control, or the functioning of a stoma.
4. They must know and be able to apply appropriately the strategies which will enable them to break bad news, disentangle collusion, challenge denial, defuse anger, handle despair, develop a dialogue with a withdrawn patient, and help patients and relatives manage uncertainty.
5. They will need to relinquish their distancing tactics but are only likely to do this if they are trained in the relevant knowledge and skills and are given ongoing support, psychological and psychiatric backup.
6. A critical aspect of their role is their ability to provide effective feedback to the clinician about problems their patients are experiencing. They must do this in a way that leads clinicians to heed and act on what they say and enhances their credibility. So, they need the skills of advocacy.

Training Method

Several comments appear essential, including: the provision of detailed handouts describing the areas to be covered and the skills to be used; the demonstration of key interviewing, assessment and counselling skills by videotape; and subsequent practice with patients and relatives followed by systematic audio or videotape feedback of performance [6].

Once basic skills are mastered, the specialist nurse or social worker needs to work through the various difficult counselling situations they encounter during their practice sessions with real patients. Contrary to expectation, most patients are willing to permit recording of the nurse's or social worker's sessions with them, since they see the point of trying to improve the communication and counselling skills of health professionals. For this training to be effective, regular weekly supervision is required from someone well versed in the skills being taught, until they reach criterion. The criterion is that they recognise most (90% or more) of the problems that are present in their patients and can formulate an appropriate plan of action.

Effects of Training

The key test of this approach to improving recognition is how well such specially trained specialist nurses and social workers accurately identify, manage or refer patients with psychological and social morbidity. This was first assessed in a controlled study in which 152 patients were randomly allocated to routine care or routine care plus counselling and regular monitoring by a specially trained nurse [2]. Seventy-six percent of those patients who developed an affective disorder or a sexual or body-image problem in the first year after mastectomy were recognised and referred for help by the specialist nurse, compared with only 15% of patients so affected in the control group. Importantly, this led the monitored group to have four times less psychological morbidity than the control group. Physical and social problems were also more often effectively recognised and managed in the monitored group [7]. However, this form of monitoring had several disadvantages.

Regular coverage of psychological areas through two-monthly home visits caused some patients to worry more than they would otherwise have done. Patients looked to the nurses to help them with problems related to their disease and surgery. Other doctors and nurses looked increasingly to the specialist nurses to deal with all psychological and social problems and become even more distanced from them. The nurse or social worker charged with this monitoring role was then faced with a growing load of patients with psychological morbidity. Such a load is likely to lead to "burnout" and rapid turnover of staff.

Given these findings, it was decided to compare this regular monitoring approach with two alternatives: first, with a scheme where the specialist nurse limited her monitoring to one home visit after discharge. She then put the onus on patients who had no problems at that assessment to contact her subsequently; second, with a scheme that relied on training ward and community nurses in the required assessment skills. One hundred and eighty seven patients were allocated at random to one of these three arms [7]. There was also a control group which comprised eligible patients who could not participate in the main trial. The rates of recognition and referral of those with psychological and social morbidity were as high in the group receiving limited monitoring as in those seen every two months by a specialist nurse. They were much higher than in the group monitored by the ward staff and the control group [7]. Consequently, psychological and social morbidity was significantly reduced. Therefore, monitoring each patient by a home visit within a month after discharge proved as effective as regular monitoring every two months. Moreover, it showed that, providing patients had been assessed by such a specialist nurse on one occasion, they could be relied on to contact the nurse if problems arose later. Thus, psychological and social problems can be recognised early and lead to prompt and effective action. However, this study revealed important differences in performance between two specialist nurses who had been trained identically to the same criterion. A better recognition and referral rate was associated with extroversion, the presence of someone at home in whom the nurse could confide, prompt disclosure of concerns about patients, maintaining face-to-face contact with patients, utilisation of offered supervision and support and a previous course in oncology nursing. This means that nurses and social workers who take on this monitoring role need to be selected carefully and supervised regularly. Supervision should take the form of weekly or fortnightly meetings with a psychiatrist or clinical psychologist, during which the specialist workers can present patients they are concerned about. The use of small cassette tape recorders to record some of the consultations allows the consultations to be replayed and discussed within the supervision sessions. It also permits the supervisor to audit performance over time. As well as such feedback on offered patients, the supervisor should check at random how other patients are progressing by asking the specialist nurse or social worker about their progress and by discussing the nature (home visit or clinic visit versus telephone call), function (assessment versus counselling) and outcome of any contact with the patient or relative.

The supervisor must ensure that the specialist nurses or social workers carrying out this monitoring role are given prompt backup when they are especially concerned about a patient. Thus, if a nurse is concerned that a patient has become very depressed and may be suicidal, she knows that this patient will be seen quickly by the supervisor or psychiatric colleague. When problems are detected but are less urgent, the specialist worker will notify the treating clinician and discuss what action should be taken. Specialist workers appear to find this monitoring aspect of their role rewarding.

Without special training and the provision of regular supervision, audit and support, it is unlikely that a specialist nurse or social worker would secure and maintain a high rate of recognition of psychological and social morbidity. Instead, it is likely that she would retreat to using distancing tactics and restrict her focus to physical aspects of care.

What Kind of Specialist Worker?

In Manchester we have relied on generally trained nurses who had a good professional experience of cancer nursing. We did this because, in our early studies, patients and relatives said they would have welcomed the opportunity to talk to someone about their concerns. Ideally, that person would work closely with their specialist and have a good knowledge of cancer and cancer treatment. Such a person was likely to be a nurse since they did not perceive social workers to have sufficient medical knowledge to answer their questions. However, specialist social workers or psychiatric nurses who ensured they gained sufficient knowledge and experience of cancer care are also likely to be effective in this key monitoring role. Unfortunately, many specialist nurses and social workers are still being put into counselling posts without the required training. Therefore, it is not surprising that in many centres much of the psychological and social morbidity remains hidden.

REFERENCES

1 Maguire GP, Lee EG, Bevington DJ, Kucheman CS, Crabtree RJ and Cornell CR: Psychiatric problems in the first year after mastectomy. Br Med J 1978 (1):963-965

2 Maguire P, Tait A, Brooke M, Thomas C and Sellwood R: Effect of counselling on the psychiatric morbidity associated with mastectomy. Br Med J 1980 (281):1454-1456

3 Stewart F, Maguire P, Walker A: Psychiatric morbidity in women with cancer of the cervix. Report to Cancer Research Campaign, London 1989

4 Rosser J and Maguire P: Dilemmas in general practice: the care of the cancer patient. Soc Sci Med 1982 (16):315-322

5 Maguire P: Barriers to psychological care of the dying. Brit Med J 1985 (291):1711-1713

6 Maguire P, Roe P, Goldberg D, O'Dowd T, Jones S, Hyde C: The value of feedback in interview training for medical students. Psych Med 1978 (8):695-704

7 Maguire P, Brooke M, Tait A, Thomas C and Sellwood R: The effect of counselling on physical disability and social recovery after mastectomy. Clin Onc 1983 (9):319-324

8 Wilkinson S, Maguire P and Tait A: Life after breast cancer. Nursing Times 1988 (84):34-37

Psychological and Psychiatric Interventions

Peter Maguire

Cancer Research Campaign, Psychological Medicine Group, Christie Hospital, Manchester M20 9BX, United Kingdom

Patients with cancer and their relatives have to surmount several key hurdles if they are to adapt psychologically. Failure to manage these hurdles leads to problems which need to be resolved if more serious psychiatric morbidity is to be avoided.

Common Problems

Managing Uncertainty

A patient's fear of recurrence may be realistic. Therefore, it is important that the clinician treating the cancer acknowledge and legitimise this.

Doctor	You're right. I don't know how long you have. That's the trouble. It is uncertain. I guess this uncertainty is making it hard for you.
Patient	Yes, it is. I wish I knew where I was in terms of if and when my cancer is going to come back.

The doctor should next check if the patient would like to know what signs and symptoms could indicate a recurrence.

Doctor	What I can do, but only if *you* wish it, is to tell you what changes would indicate that your illness is back.
Patient	I would like to know.
Doctor	I think you'll start feeling very weak again. You may go off your food and find you are getting breathless.
Patient	As before then?
Doctor	Yes, but of course you are clear of any disease at the moment. So long as none of these signs are evident you should be o.k.

The patient should then be asked how often he would like to be checked to see if he is still disease-free. The doctor should add "If any of these signs should occur or anything else untoward happens between these checkups, please get in touch directly." Few relatives or patients abuse this offer.

Sometimes, the uncertainty has several components. Each component should be teased out before giving any advice.

Doctor	You say it's the uncertainty of it all. What particularly are you concerned about?
Hospice patient	Dying in pain, dying alone and being a burden to you all.
Doctor	Any other worries?
Patient	No.
Doctor	Well, that's why you are here. So that we can try to improve your pain control and get you more active. We'll do our best to ensure that you won't be on your own when it comes to it.

Breaking Collusion

Relatives usually withhold the truth because they cannot bear to cause anguish to their loved one. Therefore, the first step is to explore their reasons and indicate that you respect these for the relatives could be right. It is then important to determine what effect the collusion is having on the relatives' emotional state ("What effect has this been having on you?") and relationship with the patient ("How's it been affecting your relationship with John?"). This will usually reveal that the relative feels under great strain emotionally and is upset about not being as close to the patient. When these costs are clarified, most relatives will see the sense of considering an alternative approach to collusion.

One alternative [1] involves asking the relative to allow you to talk alone with the patient on condition that you will *not* tell him his diagnosis. Instead, you will try to establish his awareness by asking "How do you feel things are going?" The patient's reply will usually indicate if he is aware of his predicament and is willing to talk about it ("I don't think they are going at all well - I don't think I'm going to get better from this so-called ulcer"). You can then acknowledge and clarify the cue "So-called ulcer". For example:

Doctor	Why do you say "so-called ulcer"?
Patient	They've tried to kid me it's an ulcer but it's not, it's cancer.

This confirms that the patient is aware. You should then confirm that he is right and explore his feelings and concerns before seeking his permission to convey his awareness to his wife. You can then check if the couple are willing to discuss their resulting concerns with you. This is emotionally painful to do but allows a couple to identify key concerns and discuss possible solutions.

Stigma

When patients feel stigmatised by their disease it is important to check if their feelings are legitimate or represent an inappropriate response. Thus, a mother of a child with leukaemia was ostracised by her next-door neighbours who also had young children. They refused to allow their child to have any contact with the young patient. Thus, the mother's feeling that "it was as though her child had leprosy" was valid. However, a woman with cervical cancer had both rational ("They say it's caused by a virus - I think I'm contagious") and illogical views ("I'm sure every one will think I have been promiscuous"). It was possible to discuss current viral theories with her and reassure her that she was not "contagious". Her worry about other people's view of her was tackled using a cognitive approach in which her inappropriate attitudes, their antecedents, cognitive and behavioural consequences were analysed and challenged. She was then invited to substitute a positive view like, "If I talk to my friends I will find they are sympathetic" and given encouragement to test this out first with close friends and then with other friends.

Search for Meaning

Here, patients feel anguished because they cannot find an acceptable explanation for their disease or are wrongly implicating their personality, inability to handle stress, or other people. Careful exploration of their beliefs and their origins should enable them to be challenged constructively. If no adequate explanation can be found, this should be acknowledged, for example "No, I agree, I can't explain why you should have got cancer at this time" and the patient encouraged to express the consequent feelings.

When a person's religious beliefs are threatened, they may benefit from talking with a priest or chaplain.

Loss of Control

Some patients feel there is nothing they can do to help fight their disease and they can then become "helpless". They should be helped to adopt more constructive responses such as positive self-instruction ("I'll fight my cancer), healthier diet, taking more exercise and learning self-help techniques such as positive imaging, relaxation [2] and meditation.

Body Image Problems

It is important to check the nature and extent of any problems including loss of body integrity, heightened self-consciousness and loss of attractiveness as well as establishing the degree of avoidance of looking at the affected body part.

Teaching patients to relax using progressive muscular relaxation, followed by graded exposure to looking at the affected part, is usually successful and, where appropriate, a partner can be involved later. However, some patients reject this because they cannot accept themselves as they now are. They argue they are no longer acceptable as people and marked social withdrawal may be evident. A more intensive cognitive therapy approach can be helpful [3].

The patient is first taught progressive muscular relaxation and how to summon up positive images. She then learns to monitor her feelings and behaviour so that she can identify psychological, emotional and cognitive signs of anxiety and employ relaxation and imaging to eradicate them.

Then she is helped to identify negative attitudes and behaviours (for example, refusal to look at her chest wall), which are a consequence of surgery. She is encouraged to challenge the assumptions on which these attitudes and behaviours are based and to find positive self-statements to replace them ("If I let my husband see me he will hate me" versus "I am sure he loves me just as much"). She is helped to distinguish irreversible changes (breast loss) from reversible ones (avoiding looking, avoiding going out) and challenge the rationality of her behaviour.

Finally, she is encouraged to determine which reversible changes she wants to correct and to set a series of manageable goals. Each step is then rehearsed within a session before being practised as homework. She is encouraged to praise herself for each success and realise she is now beginning to resolve her problem by her own efforts.

Patients who refuse or fail to respond to these psychological approaches can benefit greatly if reconstructive surgery is possible. They must want it for themselves and be made aware of the possible pitfalls and complications.

Conditioned Responses

Here, the patient is becoming increasingly fearful because any stimulus which reminds him of chemotherapy, for example, the journey to the hospital or the sight of the chemotherapy unit, causes him to feel sick or to vomit. It is important to treat this conditioning promptly.

Burish and colleagues found that the severity of nausea and vomiting during and after chemotherapy is reduced by teaching patients relaxation techniques and positive imaging early on [4] and encouraging them to practise these methods between treatments.

Hypnotherapy combined with relaxation also appears effective [5]. The hypnotherapist suggests that the ability to relax will improve with practice, and the patient will achieve a greater degree of control over how he feels and be more able to cope with chemotherapy.

When conditioned responses worsen, it may be necessary to cover each infusion with oral Lorazepam for a few days beforehand. Infusions of Lorazepam should be used when conditioning is severe and there is a high risk that the patient will opt out of a potentially lifesaving treatment.

Psychiatric Disorders

In the absence of or despite such early intervention, psychiatric disorders may still arise and require treatment.

Depressive Illness

A depressive illness should be considered when the patient or relative complains of feeling significantly more miserable, low, or depressed than usual, this mood change has persisted for two weeks or more, been present most of the time and the patient or relative has not been able to pull themselves out of it or be distracted by friends and relatives. Most people so affected are aware of this shift from their usual mood and are perplexed by it.

For a diagnosis to be made, four or more other symptoms are required, including: repeated or early morning waking; loss of weight and appetite; impaired concentration and/or attention; problems in making decisions; feelings of hopelessness; irritability; feelings of guilt or unworthiness; inability to enjoy life; loss of interest; and finding it an increasing effort to cope with day-to-day chores. When cancer is present, symptoms that could be due to it rather than to depression (like loss of appetite and weight) should be ignored in arriving at a diagnosis).

The illness should be treated once it is clear that it is a persisting reaction and even earlier than two weeks if the mood change is severe and/or there is any suicidal risk. It will usually respond to antidepressant medication in adequate dosage within 4 to 6 weeks. It is important to choose an antidepressant with minimal side effects, since most patients are treated as outpatients and are afraid these drugs will sedate them and impair their daily functioning. There is also a danger that they will wrongly attribute side effects to spread or recurrence of the disease. Newer antidepressants like Dothiepin (Prothiaden), Lofepramine (Gamanil) and Trazadone (Molipaxin) are usually well tolerated, relatively free of side effects and effective.

If a patient with a depressive illness is also very anxious or agitated, a sedating tricyclic antidepressant like amitryptiline (Tryptizol) is to be preferred. If they are ruminating about their disease, Chlomipramine (Anafranil) is helpful. Patients who are retarded by their depression will benefit from an alerting tricyclic antidepressant like Imipramine (Tofranil). If agitation continues despite the use of a sedating antidepressant, a neuroleptic drug like Thioridazine (Melleril) or Chlorpromazine (Largactil) should be added.

Tricyclic antidepressants should not be used in patients with heart disease, prostate disease or glaucoma and given, if at all, in limited amounts to patients at risk of suicide.

When prescribing antidepressant medication, it is important to make several points to the patient or relative, otherwise they may stop it prematurely or refuse to take it.

Give a Rationale for the Depressive Illness

Explain that depression is a well-recognised and common illness which is known to be caused by exposure to stressful life events. The stress triggers a biochemical change which results in a depletion in certain chemicals called amines. This depletion causes the depression.

Explain Treatment

So, a drug is needed to correct this depletion. Antidepressants have this specific action. It is necessary to prescribe one because you have already explained that despite your best efforts you have been unable to fight your way out of your depression.

Explain the Advantages and Disadvantages of Antidepressant Therapy

Emphasise that the drug does not cause dependence and that the patient should be able to stop it without difficulty when the time comes. This will usually be within 4 to 6 months of starting. Stopping medication earlier carries a high risk that the depression will recur.

Explain what the side effects might be, the precautions to be taken with alcohol, driving and machinery, and the action to be taken if problems arise.

Finally, make it clear that once the mood has begun to lift, you will help the patient or relative resolve any other problems they require help with. Otherwise, they may feel they are being offered drugs as a substitute for real psychological help.

Electroconvulsive therapy (ECT) accelerates recovery from depression and is most effective in those patients who are so depressed that their thinking becomes impaired. They can then develop false but unshakeable beliefs (delusions) as in the following example. Contraindications to ECT include a history of a recent stroke, myocardial infarct or brain metastases.

Mrs. W was a 50-year old housewife who became severely depressed after undergoing mastectomy and radiotherapy. Despite being found to be disease-free, she became convinced that her body was rotting away and that cancer was "eating her up". She saw no point in eating as she was convinced she was dying. She was started on amitryptiline to forestall relapse in the longer term and given a course of ECT. She made a complete recovery after 8 ECT treatments (given at a rate of 2 a week). ECT should also be considered if there is a high suicidal risk since it takes a few weeks for antidepressants to work. However, suicide is not common in patients with cancer since most of those who become depressed do so because of a fear of premature death. Even so, suicidal risk must be assessed in any depressed patient.

The majority of patients with cancer and relatives who develop depression can be treated as outpatients or by their general practitioners. Admission to a psychiatric ward will only be necessary when the patient is at risk of suicide, can no longer cope with simple chores, or is providing too great a burden for the family.

It is important to treat depression in patients with recurrent or advanced disease as aggressively as in those who are disease-free, for depression seriously impairs quality of life and lowers the threshold at which physical symptoms like pain are experienced. It also causes the patient to withdraw into himself. Therefore, key areas of "unfinished" business may remain and hinder resolution of the relative's grief as well as cause a "stormy death".

Once treatment has begun to work, you can attend to any provoking factors that remain unresolved (see Common Problems) and/or are helping maintain the depression.

Cognitive therapy may be used to treat depression of moderate degree without the help of antidepressant medication, but the combination of antidepressants with cognitive therapy is probably more effective in the longer term when further provoking factors like recurrence of disease or adverse effects of treatment are probable. Rigorous clinical trials are needed to determine the exact contributions of antidepressant medication, cognitive therapy and emotional support.

Anxiety States

An anxiety state should be considered when patients or relatives complain that they feel persistently on edge, tense, are unable to relax, and cannot distract themselves or be distracted out of these feelings. They also complain of at least four other symptoms, including an inability to get off to sleep, panic attacks, autonomic symptoms (such as palpitations, sweating, headache and tremor), irritability and poor concentration.

It is crucial to make the diagnosis on the basis of the presence of these signs and symptoms to avoid dismissing anxiety as an understandable reaction which requires no treatment.

When a patient or relative is seriously disorganised by their anxiety, an anxiolytic (such as a benzodiazepine) is required for 3 to 4 weeks.

Patients should also be offered anxiety management techniques such as relaxation, imaging and distraction, and given homework exercises. They can then learn that they can identify and control their own anxiety and will avoid becoming dependent on benzodiazepines.

Aprazolam is said to be especially useful in patients who have both anxiety and depression. Clinical trials are needed in cancer patients to clarify its role.

When other problems remain, such as fear of recurrence or difficulties with body image, these should be treated.

When the anxiety state is of moderate severity, anxiety management training may be sufficient.

Cancer Phobias

Patients who are disease-free but are plagued repeatedly by fears that their cancer has returned, require and may benefit from prompt help. This should include anxiety management training, a cognitive approach to help them distinguish rational from inappropriate worries, and a programme to help them resist repeated urges to carry out self-examination or consult doctors.

Illness Behaviour

Some cancer patients fail to recover psychologically and socially despite being free of disease and off treatment [6]. They cannot believe that they have recovered and may have learned that they get more concern from others through "being ill". The value of intervention in this group, particularly behavioural programmes, remains to be evaluated.

Sexual Problems

It is important to exclude anxiety, depression, treatment-induced hormone depletion and surgical destruction of neurological pathways before attempting psychological methods. Body image problems are associated with a high incidence of sexual problems. Resolving the body image problem may result in a full sexual recovery.

The Masters and Johnson Conjoint therapy approach is usually effective but depends on the willingness of both partners to participate [7].

Role of Psychotherapy

Supportive Psychotherapy

So far, behavioural and pharmacological methods have been emphasised. But most cancer patients who develop problems can benefit from supportive therapy. This helps them identify and express their concerns and feelings and to mobilise and apply coping strategies which have helped them manage past difficulties. Thus, someone who has coped well in the past by distraction should be encouraged to use it again.

Insight-Directed Therapy

The use of short or longer-term psychotherapy as a means of helping patients modify aspects of their behaviour and personality has been advocated in the belief that it will render them less vulnerable to recurrence and could enhance survival. These claims have yet to be proved within adequate clinical trials.

Who Should Intervene?

Many of the common problems discussed could be dealt with by specialist nurses or social workers, providing they have had the relevant training. If they have also been trained in behaviour therapies, they could give the required sex therapy, anxiety management training, or cognitive therapy. However, these treatments will usually necessitate referral to a clinical psychologist or psychiatrist.

When anxiolytic, antidepressant or neuroleptic medication is required, a medical referral will be necessary. The general practitioner or treating clinician could treat much of the anxiety and depression which present, provided they use an adequate dosage, monitor progress, and are aware of the need to resolve any provoking and maintaining factors. However, if patients or relatives fail to respond, psychiatric referral is indicated, as it is with severe anxiety states or severe depressive illness.

As yet, too few psychiatrists or clinical psychologists are willing to respond promptly and helpfully to such referrals. More attention needs to be paid to training them in such liaison work within their higher professional training and to encouraging them to provide a prompt and effective backup.

REFERENCES

1 Maguire P and Faulkner A: How to communicate with cancer patients. 2. Handling uncertainty, collusion and denial. Br Med J 1988 (297):972-974

2 Bridge LR, Benson P, Pietroni PC, Priest RG: Relaxation and imagery in the treatment of depression. Br Med J 1988 (297):1169-1172

3 Tarrier N, Maguire P and Kincey J: Locus of control and cognitive therapy with mastectomy patients: a pilot study. Br J Med Psychol 1983 (36):265-270

4 Burish T, Carey M, Krozely M and Greco F: Conditioned side effects induced by cancer chemotherapy: prevention through behavioural treatment. J Consult Clin Psychol 1987 (55):42-48

5 Walker LG, Dawson AA, Pollet SM, Ratcliffe MA and Hamilton L: Hypnotherapy for chemotherapy side effects. Br J Exp Clin Hyp 1988 (5):72-82

6 Devlen J, Maguire P, Phillips P, Crowther D and Chambers H: Psychological problems associated with diagnosis and treatment of lymphomas: 2 Prospective study. Br Med J 1987 (295):955-957

7 Masters W and Johnson J: Human Sexual Inadequacy. London, Bantam Books 1970

III. Psychosocial and Behavioural Factors in Cancer Risk and Survival

Psychosocial Risk Factors in Cancer

C. Hürny

Medical Department C.L. Lory, Inselspital Bern, Freiburgstrasse, 3010 Bern, Switzerland

At first glance, there is little connection between cancer and the mind. As doctors with a mainly scientific training, we are used to considering malignant neoplastic lesions in biological terms, especially since malignant cells grow more or less autonomously and characteristically escape the control mechanisms of the body. However, on closer examination, multifactorial interactions can be discerned. These are quite evident once the diagnosis "cancer" has been made: when the patient must be informed about a fatal danger, a mutilating operation, or must withstand aggressive radiotherapy or chemotherapy, or when curative therapy is no longer to be considered, and when we have the difficult task of attending the fatally ill individual.

However, psychosocial factors may play a decisive role immediately before the establishment of the diagnosis. In a retrospective study on 200 patients with colorectal carcinoma in Britain, an average delay of 8.25 months from the occurrence of the first symptoms up to diagnosis was found. Roughly half of this delay time was to be ascribed to the patients and the other half to the family doctor [1]. The specific reasons for this behaviour of patient and physician are not clear. Lack of knowledge, unconscious avoidance of frightening information, fear of mutilation on the part of the patient and doctor are specified in the literature as the presumed reasons [2].

I wish to go even further back into the biography of the cancer patient and raise the question as to whether stressful events and privations or personality factors (to put it globally, psychosocial stress) precede the manifestation of cancer and may possibly influence the genesis and aetiology. The question is not new. The Roman doctor Galen already observed that women with a melancholy temperament have an elevated rate of breast cancer. Preeminent doctors of the modern period, e.g., Paget, Ewing and Leriche, noticed stressful circumstances of life and particular character traits in their cancer patients [3]. In 1983, Snow investigated 250 unselected cancer patients at the London Cancer Hospital. In most of these patients, he found severe psychological stress, difficulties at work, or mechanical traumas which were related in time with the manifestation of the cancer. Only 19 patients did not display any special features. On the basis of this retrospective study, Snow raised the question as to whether the cancer disease had a "neurotic cause" in the majority of the cases [4].

Case Report

In 1944, Mrs. M. was born as the illegitimate daughter of a seamstress. She did not know her father. Five years later, the mother married an alcoholic. Troubled by serious problems, the mother began to beat her daughter every day. At the age of eight, the girl was moved to an unmarried foster mother, where she was well looked after but had to work hard. She did an apprenticeship in tailoring. In puberty, she had serious quarrels with her foster mother. The patient had early, multiple and unsatisfactory sexual relationships. She had to marry an Italian bricklayer at the age of 22. Two children were born. The husband was pathologically jealous and battered his wife from the very beginning. Besides her household work, Mrs. M. worked hard as a cleaning lady to supplement the family's income, but she had to hand over her entire pay to the husband. After 14 years of an agonising marriage, the patient decided to get a divorce. In order to earn enough money for herself and the two adolescent children, she accepted a job as a concierge and continued to work as a cleaning lady. She felt alone, helpless and hopeless. One year later, intermenstrual bleeding began, and inoperable cervix carcinoma was diagnosed after a further 6 months. At the first oncological examination, the patient gave the impression of being rigid and inflexible with regard to her emotional life. She could hardly express her feelings, had become socially isolated and was leading a secluded life with her two children.

In this life situation and in view of the previous history of the patient, we would not be surprised if severe depression, drug or alcohol abuse, psychogenic pain or an episode of duodenal ulcer had developed. However, we have difficulties in understanding the manifestation of a carcinoma resulting from a life situation. Although cancer originates within us, as a rule we experience it as a dire misfortune coming from the outside.

In spite of very intensive research, the causes of malignant neoplastic processes are only partly known today. Most cancer therapies are empirical. It is relatively improbable that the disease can be attributed to a single factor. According to the present state of knowledge, a multifactorial genesis must be assumed. I have summarised the aetiological factors established for individual tumours today in Figure 1 and indicated two different modes of action of psychosocial factors:

1. Indirect psychosocial factors: A certain human behaviour that is mostly complex leads to increased carcinogen exposure, e.g., smoking to lung cancer; exposure to the sun to melanoma; first sexual intercourse at early age, large number of sexual partners to cervical cancer; alcohol consumption, liver cirrhosis to liver cell carcinoma; alcohol plus smoking to cancers of the upper alimentary tract.
2. Direct psychosocial factors: Psychological stress, e.g., loss of the spouse, leads to somatic changes, for example in the immune system or in the endocrine system via psychological processes, e.g., grief in bereavement. A functional disorder, e.g., of the lymphocytes, favours the development of a malignant neoplastic lesion.

In the following I shall examine the possible modes of action of direct psychosocial risk factors in rather more detail. In order to be able to do this, I must first of all make some methodological remarks on research, which is not entirely satisfactory in this field.

Methodological Problems

The question as to direct psychosocial risk factors for cancer, i.e., with regard to direct causal relationships between psychosocial variables and cancer, is, in principle, an epidemiological problem. Epidemiological studies establish risk factors, i.e., contributory aetiological explanations. The entire variance is hardly ever explained by a single factor. In the 1960s, individual researchers believed that the genesis of cancer could be adequately and comprehensively explained by a psychosocial theory [5,6]. The idea of regarding cancer as a regressive attempt of regeneration at the biol-

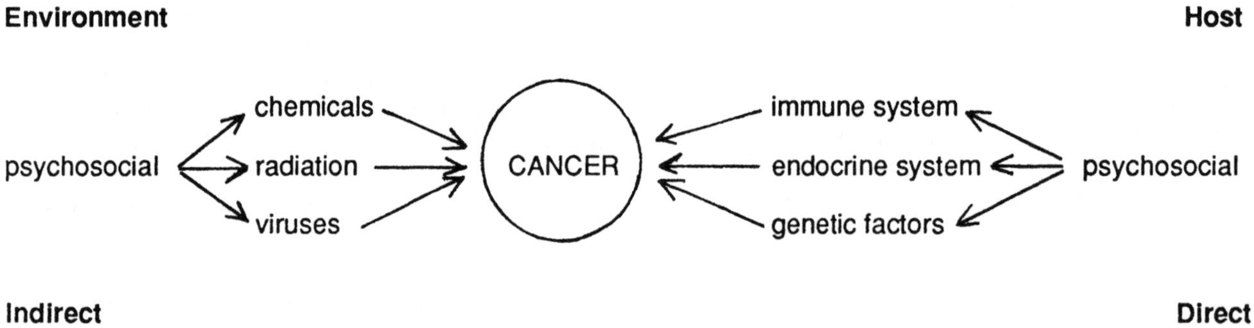

Fig. 1. Multifactorial carcinogenesis

ogical level in exhaustion or blockade of the possibilities of psychological expression is one-sided and shows a lack of understanding of the biological complexity of the problem [3].

The following general epidemiological criteria also apply to the appraisal of studies of psychosocial risk factors in cancer (Table 1).

Table 1. Epidemiological criteria for the appraisal of studies of psychosocial risk factors*

1.	Random sample
2.	Strength of association
3.	Temporal sequence
4.	Reproducibility and consistency
5.	Persistence
6.	Dose-effect relation
7.	Specificity
8.	Biological plausibility

* according to Morrison and Paffenbarger [7]

1. Random sample. Cancer is probably not a single disease process, but a collective term for the most diverse diseases. A basalioma of the skin is hardly comparable to acute myeloid leukaemia, although both are based on a histologically defined malignant neoplastic process. Psychosocial studies frequently comprise patients with various primary tumours in different stages. Furthermore, it must be borne in mind that the term "cancer" engenders sinister notions in us in a manner quite unlike any other disease. Control groups with comparable diseases are difficult to find. The existential experience of the disease may simulate or alter preexisting psychosocial factors. One hypothesis is, for example, that cancer patients have a tendency to deny or repress feelings, and that this tendency has a preexisting and causal relationship with the cancer disease [6]. Even on the basis of a well-controlled retrospective study, it is impossible to determine whether a tendency to denial and repression is a specific reaction to having cancer, or whether this tendency had been present beforehand.

2. Strength of association. The disease must be statistically associated with the factor under discussion, i.e., the factor should be substantially more frequent or rarer in a group with the disease than in a comparable control group without it. The more pronounced the association, the greater the probability that it is causal.

3. Temporal sequence. The causal factor under discussion must occur before the disease. At first glance, this appears to be trivial. However, if we consider that a neoplasm becomes clinically manifest when it consists of 10^9 cells, it must be assumed that a malignant tumour is latently present for a long time before. From the doubling time of a neoplasm, the time of the beginning of the malignant proliferation can be approximately inferred. Depending on the type of cancer, this is between 3 and 10 years before the manifestation of cancer [8]. Causal psychological factors should thus as a rule have been present for a long time in the past.

4. Reproducibility and consistency. The correlation found must be reproducible, i.e., it must be found by different investigators in different patient populations, at different times and in different places. This is problematical in some cases, since various investigators have used different instruments that are difficult to compare in the registration of psychosocial factors. The findings should be consistent with the generally known facts of the natural history and biology of the disease (cancer). Moreover, they should be consistent by age, race and demographic characteristics.

5. Persistence. The correlation must persist when other variables known as risk factors are eliminated or controlled. In lung cancer, for example, a direct psychosocial risk factor found would have to be checked to see whether it has a connection with smoking or whether it is independent.

6. Dose-effect relation. The risk of disease has to be greater in "increased exposure". The more pronounced the psychosocial characteristics, the higher the risk of cancer should be.

7. Specificity. The risk factor under discussion must be specific for the disease investigated. In our case, it would have to be specific for cancer or indeed for a specific cancer disease and not play a role in the genesis of other diseases.

8. Biological plausibility. The hypothetical correlation must be biologically plausible in the light of the present state of knowledge of the disease.

As can be seen from the 8 criteria specified, the stipulations of epidemiological science for the assumption of a causal correlation are very high. All these criteria are hardly ever fulfilled in the studies available today. However, methodological deficiencies are not only encountered in psychooncology, but are unfortunately ubiquitous. Methodological deficiencies also do not automatically mean that the hypotheses are wrong. Methodological deficiencies require caution in the interpretation of data, and they call for methodologically better investigations.

Hypotheses

The exploration of direct psychosocial risk factors in cancer disease has so far mainly given rise to two hypotheses:

1. Hypothesis of loss: severe personal losses lead to disorders of physical function via psychological changes. These favour the genesis or manifestation of cancer.
2. "Cancer personality": certain personality traits predispose to cancer.

This chapter cannot discuss all studies comprehensively and analyse them critically. The interested reader is referred to another article [3] for such analysis.

The following brief observations must be made here with regard to the "cancer personality": on the basis of numerous retrospective studies describing various personality traits in cancer patients, it cannot be decided whether these are preexistent or are to be regarded as a reaction to the disease. Open questions with regard to the strength of association, the temporal sequence, the reproducibility, consistency, persistence, specificity and not least the biological plausibility, force us to conclude that a cancer personality has not been proved today as a risk factor [10]. This contrasts with the type A behaviour, a personality pattern that has been established as a risk factor in coronary heart disease and which complies with the 8 epidemiological criteria specified above [9].

The development of the loss hypothesis will be described below and some typical studies will be analysed.

Loss, Bereavement and Disease

"... let me now talk to you about the things that you should avoid; that you become furious and express your rage from time to time pleases me, since this preserves the heat of nature; however, what I do not like is when you are troubled and take everything too much to heart. As the totality of physics teaches us, these are above all the causes which do the most damage to our body." (loc. cit. Le Shan and Worthington [11]). This recommendation was written by the Italian physician Maestro Lorenzo Sassoli to a patient in 1402.

Hypotheses frequently arise on the basis of clinical observations, namely the anecdotal ones. At the beginning, I referred to a patient with cervical cancer whom I examined in the outpatient clinic. This case report suggests the hypothesis that more frequent losses occur in the prior history of cancer patients (specifically cervical cancer patients). If one wants to know whether increasing losses and the later occurrence of cancer are fortuitous or whether there is a correlation, a first step is to check the observation in other patients with the same disease. This has been done on a large scale. The literature is full of case reports. For example, Le Shan frequently found severe losses in childhood with abysmal and ultimate hopelessness in the extensive psychoanalytical treatment of cancer patients with various locations of the primary tumour [12,13]. On the basis of further uncontrolled studies, he has described what he considers to be a typical development pattern for cancer patients [14]. The drama begins with the death or the definitive absence of one parent in early childhood. This leads to a feeling of having been deserted, or loneliness. In part, the child experiences this state as being his or her own fault. The child feels rejected and his or her later relationships are superficial and unstable. By trial and error he or she is later able to deepen and maintain one of these difficult relationships. A second, crucial loss of this significant reference person reactivates the old feelings of hopelessness. Months to years after this second loss, the first signs of cancer become manifest. The life history of the patient with cervical carcinoma described above fits quite exactly into this pattern.

The next step in checking the hypothesis is the retrospective controlled clinical study. The investigation of Graham et al. [15] is specified as an example. They investigated 447 patients with cervical cancer and 711 control patients with regard to traumatic events such as death of a significant reference person, divorce, unemployment, financial privations and chronic disease in the family in the 5 years before establishment of the cancer diagnosis. The control group consists of patients with another primary tumour and other chronic non-neoplastic diseases. The precise distribution of diagnoses within the control group is not specified. The cervical carcinoma patients did not show any increased incidence of losses in the 5 years before diagnosis compared to the controls. This investigation indicates that losses are not specific for patients with cervical carcinoma but does not generally preclude loss as a risk factor for cancer because of the mixed control group (patients with cancer and patients with other diseases). Moreover, only the fact of the loss and not its psychological consequences, e.g., helplessness and hopelessness, are considered. Possibly it is not the loss itself, but certain effects of the loss that give rise to the disease. We may possibly be confronted with a disease-specific, but not a cancer-specific factor. To answer this question a reference group of healthy subjects would have been necessary in this study.

Schmale and Iker [16,17] examined the possible connection of helplessness and hopelessness with manifestation of a cervical carcinoma without knowledge of histological findings. They investigated 68 women who showed stage III according to Papanicolaou in the cervical cytology in routine investigations, but who otherwise were completely healthy. In the patients who reacted with hopelessness to recent life events in the previous 6 months, a carcinoma was predicted "blindly" in the conisation biopsy to be carried out later. If the subjective emotion of hopelessness was lacking, mere dysplasia was prognosticated. A correct classification was possible in 73.6% of the cases, and was thus not random ($p \leq 0.001$). Carcinoma patients did not differ from dysplasia patients in this study with regard to losses that they actually had, but merely in their tendency to react to impending losses with hopelessness. Schmale regards the subjective emotion of hopelessness and the tendency to react with helplessness as a permissive, that is, contributory condition, not as an aetiological factor for the manifestation of a carcinoma in the presence of dysplasia.

On the basis of the selected studies quoted so far, it is difficult to determine whether losses and/or their psychological or social effects may contribute to the risk of developing cancer. Besides the replication of retrospective studies, it is logical to check the hypothesis prospectively, i.e., one should not look for losses in the previous history of cancer patients who have already developed the disease, but healthy subjects who suffer a severe loss must be followed up over years and checked as to whether increased carcinomas occur compared to subjects who did not experience a loss of this kind.

Large-scale prospective studies have been carried out on individuals who lost their spouses by death, i.e., widows and widowers. In the first weeks up to 10 years after the death of the partner, the mortality is raised 2 to 10-fold compared to controls of the same age without such a loss, especially in men [18]. The increased risk seems to have 2 peaks. Shortly after the loss (1 week to 1 year) widowed men and women have a higher mortality risk, mainly due to acute incidents of coronary heart disease. In the long term, up to 10 years after the loss of the partner, only men have a higher mortality risk [19]. An example is the large-scale American prospective study in Washington County, Maryland, carried out by Helsing and Szklo [20]. Follow-up examinations were carried out up to 1975 in 4,032 adults who had lost their spouses between 1963 and 1974 and compared with the same number of married persons. For men, the mortality in this 12-year period was raised by 1.5 to 4 times in the different age groups, except for the 75-year olds and older. In contrast to earlier studies, no difference was found for women. The "strong sex" thus appears to be weaker with regard to coping with losses. In most studies, the mortality is not raised in correlation with a specific disease, but the distribution of the causes of death corresponds to that of the general population [21].

With regard to the hypothesis that loss plays a role as an aetiological factor in cancer, the following observation can be made: the risk of dying in the years after the loss of the spouse, including the risk of dying of cancer, is raised, especially for men [22]. However, loss must be rejected as a specific risk factor for cancer, i.e., it is not more probable that one will die of cancer than of any other cause after the loss of the marriage partner.

The question now arises as to whether it is not the loss itself, but rather the way in which a person reacts to it (i.e., the nature of the grief process) that plays a role. The prospective study of Shekelle et al. [23] possibly provides a preliminary answer to this question. In 1958, 2,020 male staff members of Western Electric Co. filled in an MMPI (Minnesota Multiphasic Personality Inventory) which could be evaluated. Of those who displayed D (depressivity) as the highest value in their personality profile at that time, 2.3 times more had died of cancer in 1975 (i.e., 17 years later) than had controls ($p \leq 0.001$). This correlation was maintained when other risk factors such as age, alcohol and tobacco consumption, occurrence of cancer in the family, and work situation were eliminated statistically. A correlation was not found between a high D value and the mortality from all other diseases. At 20 years' follow up again a significant correlation between depressivity and cancer incidence and mortality was found [24]. In the prospective Walnut Creek Contraceptive Drug Study, 8,932 women completed an evaluable MMPI in 1968-1969 [25]. Up to 1982, i.e., in the 13 years after the psychological testing, 117 women got breast cancer. Besides a small but significant difference in the "lie score", these women, as compared to those remaining in good health, showed no difference in the initial MMPI profile. Neither was the D-score high, compared to the other scores of the MMPI, nor was there an absolute increase of the D-score itself. Incidence of other neoplastic diseases was not investigated. In the male subjects of the Western Electric Co. Study the association of initial high D-scores was more pronounced with cancer mortality than with cancer incidence. In the Walnut Creek Contraceptive Drug Study the (breast) cancer mortality was not investigated.

According to these investigations, a tendency to depression and, among other things, also to helplessness and hopelessness, appears to be a risk factor for later development of a malignant tumour, but only in men.

Personal loss is thus probably not a specific risk factor for cancer, but the tendency to depression (i.e., a possible way of reacting to losses) might have an effective causal connection with cancer, particularly in men but not in women.

Psychobiological Interrelationships

If it is assumed that psychosocial events and conditions, for example, personal loss and the psychological reaction to this, e.g., grief, can increase the susceptibility to somatic diseases, the question arises as to how this occurs. For example, the causal mechanisms of the raised risk of death after loss of the spouse have not been clarified. There may be environmental factors affecting the diseased persons and the surviving dependants in the same way. Social effects of the loss, e.g., isolation, neglect, lack of care and food, might play a role. A major factor is probably also the psychological adaptation to the loss. In Figure 2, I have attempted to represent possible connections between direct psychosocial risk factors and biological events. Mainly the nervous system, the hypophyseal endocrine system and the immune system are considered today as mediators between the environment, the mind and the body. Moreover, they are subject to mutual interactions. Numerous hormones, especially cortisone, adrenaline and noradrenaline, thyroxine, growth hormone, insulin and the various sex hormones, play a major role in the normal development and function of humoral and especially cell-mediated immune defense [26]. Destruction of the hypophysis leads to damage to the thymus and *vice versa* [27]. The lymphocytes possess receptors for corticosteroids, growth hormone, insulin, histamine, alpha and beta adrenergic and cholinergic receptors [3]. The interactions are multifactorial and not exactly known in detail. Nevertheless, it may be stated that complicated and complex connections are becoming apparent between mental experience and processes at the cellular level.

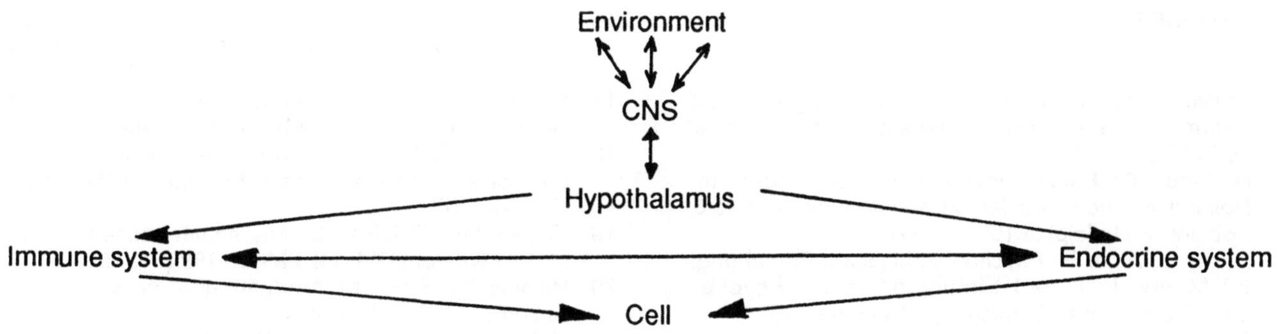

Fig. 2. Possible pathways of direct psychosocial risk factors

Finally, I should like to quote as an example the first study that shows the possible effects of personal loss on the immune system. In 1977, the group led by Bartrop [28] found a substantial attenuation of the cellular immune response (i.e., of the T-lymphocytes to mitogen stimulation) 6 weeks after the death of the partner in a well-controlled study in 26 widows and widowers. The attenuation of the T-cell function was evidently independent of hormonal factors (cortisone, prolactin, STH and thyroxine). Later investigations have reproduced these results [29] and multifarious correlations between psychosocial stress and immune function have been discovered [30-32]. However, at present there are no established biological indicators for a subtle assessment of immune function *in vivo*. All the available lymphocyte function tests are *in vitro* procedures only reliable for severe impairment of immune function (AIDS).

Conclusion

On the basis of a clinical report, the hypothesis is discussed as to whether severe personal losses or privations are a contributory risk factor to the later development of cancer with reference to selective representative investigations from the literature. It may beconcluded that severe personal losses, e.g., death of a spouse, are followed by an elevated risk of illness and death (also from cancer!), above all in men, but that the loss is not a specific risk factor for cancer. Furthermore, it can be suspected that the tendency to depression or to helplessness and hopelessness, i.e., a possible psychological response to losses, may make a specific contribution to a later manifestation of cancer, again, only in men. According to recent investigations of the correlation between psychological experience and immune function, the hypothesis would be plausible in biological terms. However, this supposition will have to be substantiated or rejected on the basis of further prospective investigations.

One must warn against precipitate conclusions, especially in the press. This may under certain circumstances result in severe insecurity of our patients. In an oversimplification, modern health apostles have equated the subjective attitude to life and to the cancer disease with the prognosis [33]. Consequently, patients often have the feeling that, if they are unable to think "positively" about the disease, it will progress rapidly. Wrongly understood interrelationships between the mind and cancer prevent adequate confrontation of the patient with his or her disease. This includes transient periods of despair and sadness.

"Happy people do not die of cancer" could be read some time ago in the tabloid press. The problem is hardly as simple as this.

REFERENCES

1 Hollyday HW, Hardcastle JD: Delay in diagnosis and treatment of symptomatic colorectal cancer. Lancet 1979 (i):309-311

2 Holland JC: Psychologic aspects of cancer. In: Holland JC and Frei E (eds) Cancer Medicine. Lea & Febiger, Philadelphia 1982 p 1176

3 Hürny C, Adler R: Psychoonkologische Forschung. In: Meerwein F (ed) Einführung in die Psycho-Onkologie. Huber, Bern/Stuttgart/Vienna 1981

4 Snow H, 1893, cit. in Baltrusch HJF: Psyche - Nervensystem - neoplastischer Prozess. Z psychosom Med 1963 (9):229; 1964 (10):1; 1964 (10):157

5 Le Shan LL: A basic psychological orientation apparently associated with malignant disease. Psychiat Quart 1961 (35):314-330

6 Bahnson CB, Bahnson MB: Cancer as an alternative to psychosis: A theoretical model of somatic and psychologic regression. In: Kissen DM, Le Shan LL (eds) Psychosomatic Aspects of Neoplastic Disease. Pitman Medical Publishing Co Ltd, New York 1964 pp 184-202

7 Morrison FR, Paffenbarger RA: Epidemiological aspects of bio-behavior in the etiology of cancer. A critical review. In: Weiss SM, Herd JA, Fox BH (eds) Perspectives on Behavioral Medicine. Academic Press, New York 1981

8 Fox BH: Premorbid psychological factors as related to cancer incidence. J Behav Med 1978 (1):45-133

9 Jenkins CD: Behavioral risk factors in coronary heart disease. Ann Rev Med 1978 (29):543-562

10 Bammer K: Krebs und Psychosomatik. Kohlhammer, Stuttgart/Berlin/Köln/Mainz 1981

11 Le Shan LL, Worthington RE: Loss of cathexes as a common psychodynamic characteristic of cancer patients. An attempt of a clinical hypothesis. Psychol Rep 1956 (2):183-193

12 Le Shan LL, Gassman ML: Some observations on psychotherapy with patients suffering from neoplastic disease. Am J Psychother 1958 (12):723-734

13 Le Shan LL: Untersuchungen zur Persönlichkeit der Krebskranken. Z psychosom Med Psychoanal 1963 (9):246-253

14 Le Shan LL: An emotional life-history pattern associated with neoplastic disease. Ann NY Acad Sci 1966 (125):780-793

15 Graham S, Snell IM, Graham JB, Ford L: Social trauma in the epidemiology of cancer of the cervix. J Chron Dis 1971 (24):711-725

16 Schmale AH, Iker H: The psychological setting of uterine cervical cancer. Ann NY Acad Sci 1966 (125):807-813

17 Schmale AH, Iker H: Hopelessness as a predictor of cervical cancer. Soc Sci Med 1971 (5):95-100

18 Jacobs S, Ostfeld A: An epidemiological review of the mortality of bereavement. Psychosom Med 1977 (39):344-357

19 Rogers MP, Reich P: On the health consequences of bereavement. N Engl J Med 1988 (319):510-512

20 Helsing KJ, Szklo M: Mortality after bereavement. Am J Epidem 1981 (114):41-52

21 Helsing KJ, Comstock GW, Szklo M: Causes of death in a widowed population. Am J Epidem 1981 (116):524-532

22 Hürny C, Holland JC: Letter to the Editor. Gen Hosp Psychiat 1983 (5):301-303

23 Shekelle RB et al: Psychological depression and 17-year risk of death from cancer. Psychosom Med 1981 (43):117-125

24 Persky VW, Kempthorne-Rawson J, Shekelle RB: Personality and risk of cancer: 20-year follow up of the Western Electric Study. Psychosom Med 1987 (49):435-499

25 Hahn RC, Petitti DB: Minnesota Multiphasic Personality Inventory - rated depression and the incidence of breast cancer. Cancer 1988 (61):845-848

26 Rogers MP, Dubey D, Reich P: The influence of the psyche and the brain on immunity and disease susceptibility. A critical review. Psychosom Med 1979 (41):147-164

27 Pierpaoli W, Sorkin E: Relationship between thymus and hypophysis. Nature (London) 1973 (246):405-409

28 Bartrop RW, Lazarus L, Mekhurst E, Kiloh LG, Penny R: Depressed lymphocyte function after bereavement. Lancet 1977 (i):834-836

29 Schleifer SJ et al: Suppression of lymphocyte stimulation following bereavement. J Amer Med Assoc 1983 (250):374-377

30 Locke SE: Stress, adaptation and immunity. Studies in humans. Gen Hosp Psychiat 1982 (4):49-58

31 Kiecolt-Glaser JK et al: Chronic stress and immunity in family casegivers of Alzheimer's disease victims. Psychosom Med 1987 (49):523-535

32 Kiecolt-Glaser JK et al: Marital quality, marital disruption and immune function. Psychosom Med 1987 (49):13-34

33 Cousins N: Anatomy of Illness. Norton, London/New York 1979

Behavioural Factors in Cancer Risk and Survival

Darius Razavi [1], Jimmie C. Holland [2]

1 Service de Médecine et Laboratoire d'Investigation Clinique H. Tagnon (Unité de Psycho-Oncologie), Institut Jules Bordet, Centre des Tumeurs de l'Université Libre de Bruxelles, 1 rue Héger Bordet, 1000 Brussels, Belgium
2 Psychiatry Service, Memorial Sloan-Kettering Cancer Center, 1275 York Avenue, New York, NY 10021, USA

The risk of cancer at a number of sites is directly related to behaviours that expose the individual to carcinogens. Since change of behaviour also represents the greatest opportunity for prevention of cancer, this area is an important aspect of psychooncology. Behaviours contribute to 50% of cancer deaths. Smoking alone accounts for about 30% of cancer deaths [1]. Oncologists can play an important role by teaching patients about smoking cessation and by serving as non-smoking models. This chapter focusses on smoking, diet, alcohol consumption, sexual practices and sun and occupational exposures, which are the habits most critical to impact. Early detection and treatment compliance are reviewed as means of secondary prevention.

Smoking as a Risk Factor

Most research has gone into understanding the primary factors in the two major aspects of smoking: initiation and maintenance.

Preventing Initiation

Smoking is most likely to be initiated in adolescence. Factors that have been found to play a role are curiosity, rebelliousness, smoking as a symbol of adulthood, social confidence and the social pressure that comes from seeing parents, siblings and peers smoke [2]. Many researchers believe that social pressure is probably a prime initiator of experimentation with cigarettes, both for children and adolescents, assisted by the media's portrayal of smoking as clever and sophisticated [3]. These characteristics do not separate, however, those who become habituated. Other attitudes and beliefs that facilitate the behaviour are the need to be better accepted by others and the belief that smoking helps in coping with stress [4].

The factors contributing to initiation explain why prevention programmes have been organised to teach children and adolescents about the hazards of smoking. Most of these programmes take place at school, although media campaigns (posters, radio, television) are also helpful. Most of the recent prevention programmes provide information about the short and long-term health consequences of smoking, as well as training (education and/or role playing sessions) in dealing with peer pressure. A significantly smaller number of children that take up smoking and increased knowledge on smoking is generally observed in pupils exposed to school-based prevention programmes [5,6]. Long-term assessment of the effectiveness of these programmes is not yet available. Efforts such as those in Scandinavia to create a smoke-free generation by focussing on young parents with young children, are now being introduced in the United States.

Some are sceptical about the effects of these interventions [7]. More active approaches have recently been proposed by the Europe-Against-Cancer programme: increased taxation on tobacco, prohibition of cigarettes with a high tar content, prohibition of tax-free tobacco sales and protection of children from tobacco sales. It is perhaps useful to recall that education is a means to prevent initiation of smoking, not a means of cessation by itself. Methods using fear-arousing education show that, although fear facilitates persuasion and strengthens the intention to quit smoking, it does not usually lead to quitting [8].

Encouraging Cessation of Smoking

The major factor in the maintenance of smoking behaviour is the development of nicotine dependence. Avoidance of withdrawal symptoms assures continuation. The degree of physical dependence is directly related to the number of cigarettes smoked daily and to their nicotine content. The symptoms of nicotine withdrawal are readily recognised by smokers: irritability, anxiety, inability to concentrate, arousal disturbances and intensified craving for a cigarette [9]. The desire for another cigarette occurs when the level of nicotine falls to a level which induces withdrawal symptoms.

There are psychosocial as well as physiological factors that affect the maintenance of smoking behaviour. These factors are explained by changes in plasma nicotine levels; the craving and smoking behaviour which follow; the high relapse rates seen in cigarette smokers even after nicotine levels have remained at zero for a long period of time; smoking responsiveness to emotional states that change rapidly; why individuals have difficulty quitting smoking when under stress; and the long developmental history of smoking [7].

Once initiated, smoking becomes a habit that can be understood by conditions of social learning. The principles of operant-conditioning and the concepts of imitation, social reinforcement and the symbolic, vicarious and self-regulatory processes, partly explain this development [10]. Smoking becomes a stable behaviour pattern marked by automatic and unconscious reaching for cigarettes and matches, and a decreasing awareness of the habit [11-13]. Smoking is also related to mood and affect, being a means to obtain pleasure or relieve unpleasantness [14,15].

Physiological, behavioural, psychological and emotional factors interact in the consolidation of smoking behaviour [7,16-19]. These concepts have all contributed to the development of behavioural interventions for smoking cessation programmes. The major smoking cessation methods utilise: drug therapy, education, behaviour modification, hypnosis, acupuncture and combinations of these [20]. Rates of immediate quitting at the end of treatment are between 40 and 90% [21,22]. However, relapse rates in most programmes are high: 40-50% relapse is seen at one year. There is a need for more randomised controlled trials that examine both short-term and long-term efficacy. Supportive techniques and counselling methods used indicate that no single technique, whether hypnosis or pharmacotherapy along with support, has emerged as most successful. Personal factors of motivation, expected benefits, good social support and even a history of prior successful cessation attempts appear to be major contributors to success.

Along with these clinical interventions, there have been large-scale programmes [23]: individuals are usually referred either to an intervention group for smoking cessation or to their usual source of medical care. In general, these investigations demonstrated that mass media approaches to smoking cessation had a minor impact. Reasons proposed as to why a mass media approach is less effective than a clinical approach in changing beliefs and behaviours are that face-to-face interventions increase the impact of information; that media messages are symbolic, abstract, and often based on guesses of what could be effective; and that the recipients of the media messages are in different situations that may contribute to either a negative or positive effect. Clearly, physicians in oncology can play an important role by introducing the need for smoking cessation with patients and relatives at the time of a cancer diagnosis, and by being outspoken advocates in their communities for smoking education.

Other Risk Factors

Excessive Alcohol Intake

Little public attention has been paid to the data that strongly associate excessive alcohol intake with cancer of several sites: mouth, pharynx, larynx, oesophagus and possibly pancreas [24]. Since heavy smoking and heavy drinking very often go together, the risk of cancer rises sharply in individuals who do both. The relative contribution of one versus the other is often hard to assess in these individuals. Data suggest that heavy intake of both has a synergistic, and not simply additive, effect on the risk. This synergistic effect raises the relative risk of oral cancer, in heavy drinkers who also smoke, up to 15 times [25]. The pathogenic mechanism hypothesised is that alcohol may act as a promotor or cofactor with tobacco acting as the initiator, thus accounting for the synergistic effect. Ethanol may act as an irritant to membranes, making them vulnerable to other carcinogens, to the adverse effects of vitamin deficiency and to malnutrition or to immune suppression. Whether alcohol acts as an irritant, as an augmentor of other carcinogens, or as a cause, through associated malnutrition, is unknown, but the data are persuasive concerning increased risk, particularly with distilled spirits (primarily whiskey). While there is less risk with wine and beer, heavy beer drinking is associated with increased risk of colon and bladder cancer. The absence of public health campaigns on the carcinogenic effects of alcohol is remarkable, given the emphasis on tobacco in this respect. While the relative number of cases annually attributed to alcohol is 2-4%, considerably below those attributed to cigarette smoking, the incidence of head and neck cancer among heavy drinkers who smoke is high. Encouraging national efforts in the U.S. are the recommendation of warnings on alcohol bottles and the limitation of alcohol advertising.

Diet

Diet has become increasingly important in understanding cancer risk, particularly with respect to high fat intake and obesity. The risk of several tumours is elevated by weight significantly above the ideal: cancer of the endometrium, breast, gall bladder, ovary, prostate and colon. Doll and Peto [1] attributed 35% of cancer deaths to increased risk by virtue of dietary factors which included both overnutrition and high-fat diet. A 1979 Cancer Society survey of deaths confirmed the risk for women [26]. However, a recent review by the National Cancer Institute of several studies noted less risk of prostate and premenopausal breast cancer, but increased risk of endometrial and postmenopausal breast cancer [27]. The cause appears to be prolonged exposure to higher levels of oestrogen stored in fat tissues, adding to postmenopausal breast and endometrial risk. Trials of reduced fat content, both as a means of reducing genetic high risk and as a means of reducing risk of recurrence in women with stage I breast cancer, are underway. The evidence appears particularly strong in relation to breast and endometrial cancer, suggesting an appropriate basis for large clinical trials on fat reduction in the diet, from the usual 40% to less than 20%. The level to which fat must be reduced is regarded by some as almost incompatible with compliance. The association of obesity with shorter survival in breast cancer as the second most significant factor after nodal status is another important indication.

Both epidemiological and animal data suggest that colon cancer is positively correlated with total dietary fat intake. The mechanism proposed is that fat in the diet enhances cholesterol and bile acid synthesis by the liver, leading to increased amounts of sterols and their metabolites in the colon, which act as promotors in colon carcinogenesis. Lipkin and Newmark [28] have found in several studies that increased proliferation of colonic epithelial cells is associated with higher cancer risk; oral calcium reversed this proliferation as well as the mitogenic effects of fatty and free bile acids by conversion to insoluble chemical compounds [28].

Fibre in the diet is also a recommended dietary change which may help reduce the risk of colorectal cancer. Increased bran cereals and whole wheat in the diet is recommended, which may act by shortening the time that stool is in the colon, or by altering possible carcinogens or bacteria in stool. Combined reduced fat intake with increased fibre is recommended.

Sexual Behaviour

Sexual mores vary with culture, as do the circumstances and the age of initiation of sexual activity. They affect cancer risk in positive and negative ways. For example, the risk of breast cancer is reduced by an early full-term pregnancy, which appears to be the result of the protective effect of a full-term pregnancy on the reduction of prolactin levels as compared to those of nulliparous women or women who have a late first full-term pregnancy [29]. A high relative risk of anal cancer has been reported in men with a history of receptive anal intercourse in homosexual relations [30]. The association of genital warts, caused by the papilloma virus, may be the cause of anal cancer in such situations.

The clearest association of sexual behaviour and cancer is that of cervical cancer, which is most common among women with a history of early sexual intercourse with multiple partners. There is a strong suggestion that cervical cancer is a sexually transmitted disease related to sexual exposure to a herpes virus carried by the man. He carries the virus by virtue of wider sexual exposures [31]. The number of sexual partners during and following adolescence is highly significant, this age being the most important period of increased risk, perhaps reflecting the period that cervical cells are most susceptible to sexually transmitted carcinogenic agents [32]j. The mortality from cervical cancer has been declining steadily in North America for the last 50 years, while precancerous cervical lesions have increased due to more cervical smears, earlier diagnosis and better hygiene. The current campaign to increase the use of condoms as a means of preventing the spread of AIDS is also the best potential preventive for invasive cervical cancer.

Sunlight Exposure

Exposure to sunlight, especially among fair-skinned individuals, is a risk factor for skin cancers primarily appearing on the exposed face, arms and hands. Older individuals, especially men who have worked outside for many years, develop basal cell and squamous cell carcinomas. This is due to ultraviolet radiation, which affects the melanin content in the cells and hence the development of deeper colour, tan and freckles. The chronic effect may be the formation of keratosis, premalignant lesions, and finally carcinoma. The role of solar exposure in the formation of melanoma is less clear, but it is a risk factor in susceptible individuals. While exposure related to outdoor work can be reduced by wearing sleaves, gloves and by covering the head, exposure to sunlight as part of the "healthy tanned look" cult is a needless risk. Education about the risk of excessive exposure, especially in southern climates and of fair-skinned vulnerable individuals, is needed. Sun screens have become highly effective and their use should be encouraged [33].

Occupational Exposures

The awareness that environmental exposures may lead to increased incidence of a particular cancer is not new - nor is procrastination in eliminating the risk. Sir Percivall Potts observed a high incidence of scrotal cancer among chimney sweeps in London and suggested it to be due to their continuously wearing soot-laden clothes without washing or bathing. It was 200 years before efforts were successful in protecting these young men. Chromates and aniline dyes have long been known to increase the frequency of certain tumours. Asbestos, used for insulation in ships, houses and schools, was found to be a substance whose fibres remain in the body and produce mesothelioma of the peritoneum and pleura, as well as lung cancer. Previously an uncommon tumour, it became more frequent following a lag of 20 to 30 years in exposed individuals and their families (exposure to workman's clothes containing asbestos fibres). Selikoff and Hammond estimated that the risk of exposed asbestos workers increased eightfold if the worker was also a heavy smoker [34]. Vinyl chloride has been shown to cause hepatoma, a primary liver tumour otherwise rarely seen.

Occupation-related carcinogens demand particular responsibility on the part of labour, management and regulatory agencies. Chemical carcinogens in industrial plants, and radioactive materials in particular, emerge as major problems for the future, as accidents may expose the adjacent community as well as plant employees. Storage and containment of radioactive waste is an increasingly difficult issue as space becomes more limited.

Early Detection

In most tumours, early detection contributes to successful treatment. Delay in seeking consultation after recognising a suspicious symptom, such as a breast mass, is associated with poor survival. When the interval between the time a symptom is first noticed and first consultation exceeds 3 months, it is defined as delay [35]. Twenty percent of women with breast symptoms were reported to delay for at least 3 months [36,37]. There are, of course, other factors that contribute to the impact of delay on survival, for example the rapidity of tumour growth.

Factors associated with early detection or delay are the specific cancer symptoms, the patient's knowledge about cancer and its treatments, and personality traits and attitudes that contribute to delay, e.g., denial of bad news, disbelief that any physical problem can be serious.

Delay can be related to the fact that cancer at an early stage does not alter everyday functioning, that symptoms often have a slow and insidious onset and development, and that symptoms are often ambiguous. Emotions may play an important role too. Fear can induce the patient to try to control the anticipated danger and to request help. This behaviour reduces the delay before consultation. In the case or breast cancer, fear may lead women to deny the danger and/or actively avoid the diagnosis of cancer and its implications. Breast Self-Examination (BSE) is an example of a highly effective means of early detection of breast cancer, since women usually are the ones who feel a lump. Educating women to examine themselves monthly has contributed to diagnosis of earlier and more curable cancers. Women are also being encouraged to have regular mammograms; this has also contributed to the increase in breast cancer diagnosis, primarily of tumours at early localised node-negative stages. BSE training programmes have been tested for their efficacy. BSE was seen to increase the possibility of early detection, but not overall participation [38]. The technique of self-examination is improved by this training, but the frequency of women who actually practice it often remains unchanged [39,40].

Compliance with Treatment

Compliance or noncompliance with medical regimens plays an important role in survival. The ability of a patient to adhere to an arduous treatment regimen is often enhanced by psychosocial support given by the oncologist and family. Noncompliance is a major problem in adolescents. One study reported that half of the patients with disseminated testicular cancer missed appointments or delayed the course of cisplatinum, vinblastine and bleomycin treatment [41]. Side effects contribute, but rebelliousness at this stage is often increasd by illness. Thirty-three percent of a paediatric leukaemia and lymphoma population did not comply with their prescribed drug treatment; the majority (60%) were adolescents [42].

Noncompliance is explained in part by the fact that cancer drug regimens are complex and often require continued and sustained commitment. Side effects and concerns about long-term effects are other factors. It is easy to understand why noncompliance is harder with medication taken by mouth at home.

Other factors associated with noncompliance are a low patient/staff ratio resulting in poorer emotional support and the constraints of informed consent, which today describes all side effects, as well as randomisation and the fact that the proposed investigational treatment may not be more effective than standard treatment [43].

Use of unorthodox treatments or self-medication is a behaviour that may interfere with compliance. Ten percent of adult cancer patients undergoing standard treatment admitted having received or receiving unorthodox therapies [44]. In recent years, alternative therapies have been more often utilised by educated, resourceful individuals seeking to use all means at their disposal to fight cancer. The great interest in mind-body connections and their role in control of tumour growth contribute to this. Guidelines on how to approach the issue of alternative treatments with patients and their families are available [45].

Patient compliance or noncompliance may in part be attributed to the physician. The physician's commitment to the therapeutic regimen and his willingness to support the patient both emotionally and physically during a period of adverse reactions may stimulate the patient's participation in the treatment process [46].

Conclusion

Cancer risk and survival may be related to behaviour in many different ways: exposure to carcinogens in the environment and behaviours that contribute to cancer prevention or early detection. Although there is sufficient evidence that behavioural factors can have a positive or negative influence on cancer risk, it is not sufficiently known which interventions are able to modify behaviour in the long term. Behavioural research therefore has an important role in the planning and implementation of cancer prevention efforts.

The behaviour most clearly related to cancer risk is smoking. Prevention programmes focussed on smoking should therefore be more widely organised and be made more effective. Psychological knowledge about the establishment and maintenance of smoking behaviour gives guidelines for encouraging young people not to smoke or to stop smoking if they do. Diet, sexual practices, sun exposure and exessive alcohol use are other factors that alter cancer risk and are amenable to changes in behaviour which reduce risk.

REFERENCES

1 Doll R and Peto R: The Causes of Cancer. Oxford University Press, Oxford & New York 1981
2 Lichtenstein E and Brown RA: Smoking cessation methods: Review and recommendations. In: Miller WR (ed) The Addictive Behaviors: Treatment of Alcoholism, Drug abuse, Smoking, and Obesity. Pergamon Press, Oxford 1980
3 Leventhal H: Changing attitudes and habits to reduce risk factors in chronic disease. Am J Cardiol 1973 (31):571-580
4 Smith GM: Personality and smoking: A review of the empirical literature. In: Hunt WA (ed) Learning Mechanisms in Smoking. Aldine, Chicago 1970
5 Evans RI, Rozelle RM, Mittlemark MB, Hansen WB, Bane AL and Harvis J: Deterring the onset of smoking in children: Knowledge of immediate psychological effects and coping with peer pressure, media pressure, and parent modeling. J Appl Soc Psychol 1978 (8):126-135
6 Tell GS, Klepp KI, Vellar OD and McAllister A: Preventing the onset of cigarette smoking in Norwegian adolescents: The Oslo Youth Study. Prev Med 1984 (13):256-275
7 Leventhal H, Meyer D and Nerenz D: The common sense representation of illness danger. In: Rachman S (ed) Contributions to Medical Psychology. Pergamon Press, Oxford 1980, Vol 2 pp 7-30
8 Leventhal H: Findings and theory in the study of fear communications. In: Berkowitz L (ed) Advances in Experimental Social Psychology (Vol 5). Academic Press, New York 1970
9 Shiffman SM: The tobacco withdrawal syndrome. In: Cigarette Smoking as a Dependence Process. NIDA Research Monograph No 23, DHEW Publication No ADM-79-800. US Government Printing Office, Washington 1979
10 Bandura A: Self-efficacy: Toward a unifying theory of behavioral change. Psychol Rev 1977 (84):191-215
11 Hunt WA and Matarazzo JD: Habit mechanisms in smoking. In: Hunt WA (ed) Learning Mechanisms in Smoking. Aldine, Chicago 1970 pp 65-106
12 Hunt WA, Matarazzo JD, Weiss SM and Gentry WD: Associative learning, habit, and health behavior. J Behav Med 1979 (2):111-124
13 Hunt WA and Matarazzo JD: Changing smoking behavior: A critique. In: Gatchel RJ, Baum A, Singer JE (eds) Handbook of Psychology and Health. Vol 1. Clinical Psychology and Behavioral Medicine's Overlapping Disciplines. Erlbaum, Hillsdale 1982 pp 171-209
14 Tomkins SS: Psychological model for smoking behavior. Am J Publ Health 1966 (56):17-20
15 Tomkins SS: A modified model of smoking behavior. In: Burgatta EF and Evons RR (eds) Smoking, Health and Behavior. Aldine, Chicago 1968
16 Solomon RA and Corbit J: An opponent-process theory of motivation. II. Cigarette addiction. J Abnorm Psychol 1973 (81):158-171
17 Solomon RA and Corbit J: An opponent-process theory of motivation. I. Temporal dynamics of affect. Psychol Rev 1974 (81):119-145
18 Solomon RA: An opponent-process theory of acquired motivation: The affective dynamics of addiction. In: Master J and Seligman M (eds) Psychotherapy: Experimental Models. Freeman WH, San Francisco 1977
19 Solomon RA: The opponent-process theory of acquired motivation: The costs of pleasure and the benefits of pain. Am Psychol 1980 (35):691-712
20 Stone S et al (Health and Public Policy Committee): Methods for stopping cigarette smoking. Ann Intern Med 1986 (105):281-291
21 Schwartz JL and Rider G: Review and evaluation of smoking control methods: The United States and Canada, 1969-1979. US Department of Health, Education and Welfare, DHEW Publication No (CDC) 79-8369, Washington 1978
22 Lando HA: A factorial analysis of preparation, aversion, and maintenance in the elimination of smoking. Addict Behav 1982 (7):143-154
23 United Nations Public Health Service: The Health Consequences of Smoking. US Department of Health, Education and Welfare, Washington 1975
24 Department of Health Education and Welfare, Public Health Service. In: Alcohol and Health. Second Special Report to the U.S. Congress 1974 (Ch. V) pp 53-67
25 Rothman K and Keller A: The effect of joint exposure to alcohol and tobacco on risk of cancer of the mouth and pharynx. J Chron Dis 1972 (25):711-716
26 Lew E, Garfinkel L: Variations in mortality by weight among 750,000 men and women. J Chron Dis 1979 (32):563-576
27 Cancer Letter: Hope for fatties: Avoirdupois may not increase risk after all. Cancer 1987 (13):7-9
28 Lipkin M and Newmark H: Effect of added dietary calcium on colonic epithelial-cell proliferation in subjects at high risk for familial colonic cancer. N Engl J Med 1985 (313):1381-1384
29 Musey VC, Collins DC, Musey IP, Martino-Saltzman D, Preedy JRK: Long-term effect of a first pregnancy on the secretion of prolactin. N Engl J Med 1987 (316):229-234
30 Darling JR, Weiss NS, Hislop TG, Maden CM, Coates RJ, Sherman KJ, Ashley RL, Beagrie M, Ryan JA and Corey L: Sexual practices, sexually transmitted diseases, the incidence of anal cancer. N Engl J Med 1987 (317) 973-977
31 Graham S, Rawls W, Swanson M and McCurtis J: Sex partners and herpes simplex type Z in the epidemiology of cancer of the cervix. Am J Epidemiol 1982 (115):729-735
32 University of Southern California Cancer Center: Barrier contraceptives prevent cervical cancer. Cancer Center Report 1987: 11,1,11
33 Levy SM: San Francisco, CA: Jossey-Bass. Behavior and Cancer 1985
34 Selikoff IJ and Hammond EC: Asbestos and smoking (editorial). J Am Med Assoc 1979 (242):458-459
35 Pack GT and Gallo JS: The culpability for delay in the treatment of cancer. Am J Cancer 1983 (23):443-462
36 Cameron A and Hinton J: Delay in seeking treatment for mammary tumours. Cancer 1968 (21):1121-1126

37 Willians EM, Baum M and Hughes LE: Delay in presentation of women with breast disease. Clin Oncol 1976 (2):327-331
38 Hobbs P, Haran D, Pendleton LL, Jones BE and Posner T: Public attitudes and cancer education. Int Rev Appl Psychol 1984 (33):565-586
39 Calnan MN, Chamberlain J and Moss S: Compliance with a class teaching B.S.E.: J Epidemiol Comm Health 1983 (37):264-270
40 Calnan M: The Health Belief Model and participation in programmes for the early detection of breast cancer. Soc Sci Med 1984 (19):823-830
41 Lazlo J, Lucas V and Huang A: Iatrogenic emesis model in cancer: Results of 120 patients treated with delta-9-tetrahydrocannabinol. In: Foster D (ed) The Treatment of Nausea and Vomiting Induced by Cancer Chemotherapy. Masson, New York 1981
42 Smith FB: The people's health 1830-1910. Croom Helm, London 1979
43 Hoagland A, Morrow G, Bennett J and Carnrike C: Oncologists' views of cancer patient noncompliance. Am J Clin Oncol 1983 (6):239-244
44 Cassileth B: After Laetrile, What? N Engl J Med 1982 (306):1482-1484
45 Holland JC, Geary NW and Furman A: Clinical implications of mind-body cancer research on patient's use of alternative cancer treatments. In: Current Concepts in Psycho-Oncology. Memorial Sloan-Kettering Cancer Center, New York 1987 pp 43-47
46 Lewis C, Linet MS and Abeloff MD: Compliance with cancer therapy by patients and physicians. Am J Med 1983 (74):673-678

IV. Methods of Assessment in Clinical Practice and Research

Screening for the Need of Psychosocial Intervention

Peter Maguire [1], Darius Razavi [2]

1 Cancer Research Campaign, Psychological Medicine Group, Christie Hospital, Manchester M20 9BX, United Kingdom

2 Service de Médecine et Laboratoire d'Investigation, Clinique H. Tagnon (Unité de Psycho-Oncologie), Institut Jules Bordet, Centre des Tumeurs de l'Université Libre de Bruxelles, 1 rue Héger Bordet, 1000 Brussels, Belgium

Screening for the need of psychosocial interventions in a cancer population is important in order to improve the quality of care in general and, more specifically, the effectiveness of treatment strategies. The fact that psychological problems or psychiatric disorders are insufficiently recognised explains the recent interest for developing simple screening techniques applied to medical settings.

The early recognition of psychological problems and/or psychiatric disorders should be differentiated from the screening of their risk factors. This differentiation is important because psychosocial oncology does not yet have the theoretical and empirical research background for the screening of risk factors for a given psychological problem or psychiatric disorder. Case findings refer more closely to what is feasible.

According to recent studies, the prevalence of psychological problems and psychiatric disorders in an oncological population is high. Paradoxically, there are few health services devoted to the treatment of these problems and disorders.

Why Screening?

Depending on the problem or disorder considered, the reasons for screening may be quite different. Guidelines by which screening can be evaluated have been outlined by the WHO [1]:

1. The condition must have a significant effect on the quality or quantity of life.
2. The incidence of the condition must be sufficient to justify the cost of screening.
3. The condition must have an asymptomatic period during which detection and treatment significantly reduce morbidity and mortality.
4. Treatment in the asymptomatic phase must yield a therapeutic result superior to that obtained by delayed treatment until symptoms appear.
5. Acceptable methods of treatment must be available.
6. Tests that are acceptable to patients must be available at a reasonable cost to detect the condition in the asymptomatic period.

In oncology there are, among others, three conditions in particular that could benefit from early detection: Adjustment Disorders, Anxiety Disorders and Major Depressive Disorders. The reasons are that not only do they have a significant negative effect on the quality of life, but their incidence is sufficient to justify the cost of screening. The most reliable estimates of the prevalence of DSM-III psychiatric disorders in an oncological population are about 32% for Adjustment Disorders and 6% for Major Depressive Disorders [2].

It could be argued at this point that the training of health care professionals may also be another way to improve early detection and recognition of psychological problems or psychiatric disorders. This is probably true, but considering that traditional standardised interviews leading to early detection are time-consuming [3,4], it would not be reasonable to assign all specialised staff to this procedure. A balance should be found between time allocated to screening on the one hand and to treatment or support on the other. The type of health care available and the skills of the health care provider are important factors affecting health policy in this area.

The fact that effective methods of treatment are available for several psychological problems and psychiatric disorders associated with cancer is another argument that justifies the cost of the development and implementation of a screening procedure. Moreover, even if there are no data available showing that early treatment may have therapeutic results superior to those obtained by delayed treatment, it is obvious that early effective treatment will have a positive effect on quality of life. For Adjustment Disorders, Anxiety Disorders and Major Depressive Disorders, screening is especially important since research is needed to develop more effective treatment methods (pharmacological and/or psychotherapeutic) in cancer patients.

The question as to whether screening for the need of psychosocial interventions may be harmful to an individual should also be considered [5]. Screening for the need of psychosocial interventions in a cancer population is certainly quite difficult when compared to other psychiatric screening.

In traditional psychiatric screening, it has been argued that the stigma of a psychiatric label may have negative consequences for the patient in terms of income [6], friendships and social interaction [7]. Moreover, referral to mental health specialists is poorly accepted by some patients [8].

For cancer patients, the same arguments fall short. Firstly, one study showed that 85% of cancer patients who reported significant emotional problems said they definitely or probably would go to a mental health professional if they were referred by a medical staff member and 72% responded positively to meeting a mental health professional together with their families [9]. These results confirm previous studies [10].

Moreover, for cancer patients it could not be argued that the stigma of a psychiatric label might have a harmful effect on a condition in which the stigma of being a cancer patient is already quite distressing and full of psychosocial consequences. It seems also that psychosocial studies are viewed by most patients as a helpful extension to their treatment [11].

How to Screen?

Are specific and sensitive screening methods available at a reasonable cost? The performance of screening methods are beginning to be studied in psychosocial oncology. Most of the methods tested have been self-administered questionnaires because standardised research interviews require time and training.

Beck's Depression Inventory [12], Zung's Self-Rating Depression Scale [13], the General Health Questionnaire [14], Hopkins' Symptom Checklist [15], the Rotterdam Symptom Checklist [16], and the Hospital Anxiety and Depression Scale [17] are the most frequently used screening methods in psychiatry for depression or for general psychopathology. These screening instruments generally take less than 15 minutes to complete and have proven to be quite acceptable to most patients. Most of these questionnaires have been tested in oncology and in primary care settings. The validity of the oral administration of some of these scales for in-patients has also been studied [18].

The orally administered questionnaire allows patients who have difficulties in writing or who have organic mental disorders to participate.

The determination of optimal cut-off points is a major issue for screening instruments. Receiver Operating Characteristic (ROC) has frequently been used because of its usefulness in decision-making related to screening models [19-23]. ROC Analysis expresses the relationship on a curve between the true-positive (sensitivity) and false-positive rates (1-specificity). The false-positive rate is usually related to the style or to other conditions with the same type of symptoms as the problem or disorder screened. False negatives result from the patient's need for social desirability, denial, or fearfulness, leading patients to underreport their problems or symptoms. The curve is a representation of the ability of the screening instrument to discriminate between "cases" and non-cases. The desired cut-off point is generally chosen in order to minimise the sum of false positive and false negative test results [24]. The optimal cut-off point on the ROC curve is generally determined by a cost-benefit analysis.

Cost and benefit should be objective. One must take into account the medical costs implicated in the decision to screen for a given condition and the benefits in terms of quality of life. The medical costs include the expenses related to the screening method and the optimal treatment of the disorders screened. The benefits derive from the improvement of quality of life for patients and their families. This issue is closely related to the effectiveness of the interventions designed for the treatment of the disorders.

Suggestions for Future Research and Conclusion

In oncology, psychological problems and psychiatric disorders are closely linked to cancer symptoms and to the consequences of the treatments (surgery, radiotherapy, chemotherapy). At this point, most of the research efforts have been focused on the screening of anxiety and depression, which are the most frequent symptoms of Adjustments Disorders and Anxiety and Affective Disorders associated with the diagnosis of cancer and its treatment and evolution. For these conditions, self-administered anxiety and depression questionnaires are methods with sufficient sensitivity and specificity that can be used for screening. The few studies that assess the performance of the screening methods report a sensitivity and specificity of around 75% [25-27].

The psychological problems and psychiatric disorders encountered in oncology are being studied in order to determine specificity and characteristics of diagnostic criteria. For these reasons, it was proposed to exclude the somatic items found in the usual psychiatric criteria proposed for Affective Disorders, in order to improve validity and reliability [28].

There are, however, other conditions such as organic mental disorders, anticipatory anxiety, anticipatory nausea and vomiting, treatment phobia, fatigue, sexual problems, alcohol or tobacco abuse, that could also be considered as symptoms or problems useful to be screened. A systematic screening approach should be organised with regard to the type of cancer and consequences of treatment.

REFERENCES

1 Wilson JMG and Jungner G: Principles and Practice of Screening for Disease. World Health Organization, Geneva 1986
2 Derogatis LR, Morrow GR and Fetting J: The prevalence of psychiatric disorders among cancer patients. JAMA 1983 (249):751-757
3 Hamilton M: The assessment of anxiety states by rating. Br J Med Psychol 1959 (32):50-58
4 Wing JK, Cooper JE and Sartorius N: The Measurement and Classification of Psychiatric Symptoms. Cambridge University Press, London 1974
5 Ford DE: Principles of screening applied to psychiatric disorders. Gen Hosp Psychiatry 1988 (10):177-188
6 Link B: Mental patient status, work and income: An examination of the effects of a psychiatric label. Am Sociol Rev 1982 (47):202-215
7 Phillips D: Public identification and acceptance of the mentally ill. Am J Pub Health 1966 (56):755-763
8 Bursztajn H, Barsky AJ: Facilitating patient acceptance of a psychiatric referral. Arch Intern Med 1985 (145):73-75
9 Houts P, Lipton A, Harvey H, Simmonds M, Cadieux R and Bartholomew M: Willingness to use mental health services by cancer patients with emotional problems. In: International Conference on Supportive Care in Oncology. Abstracts. Symedco, Princeton 1988 p 182
10 Worden JW, Weisman AD: Do cancer patients really want counseling? Gen Hosp Psychiatry 1980 (2):100-103
11 Fallowfield L: Do psychological studies upset patients? In: Holland JC, Massie MJ and Lesko LM (eds) Current Concepts in Psycho-Oncology and AIDS. Syllabus of the Postgraduate Course/ Memorial Sloan-Kettering Cancer Center, New York 1987 p 335
12 Beck AT and Beck RW: Screening depressed patients in family practice. Postgrad Med J 1972 (52):81-85
13 Zung WWK: A self-rating depression scale. Arch Gen Psychiatry 1965 (12):63-70
14 Goldberg DP: The Detection of Psychiatric Illness by Questionnaire: A Technique for the Identification and Assessment of Nonpsychotic Psychiatric Illness. Oxford University Press, London 1972
15 Derogatis DL: The SCL-90-R Administration, Scoring and Procedures Manual I. Clinical Psychometric Research, Baltimore 1977
16 de Haes JCJM, Pruyn JJA and Knipperberg FCG: Klachtenlijst voor kankerpatienten, eerste ervaringen. Ned Tijdschr Psych 1983 (38):403-422
17 Zigmond AS and Snaith RP: The Hospital Anxiety and Depression Scale. Acta Psychiatr Scand 1983 (67):361-370
18 Griffin PhT and Kogut D: Validity of orally administered Beck and Zung depression scales in a state hospital setting. J Clin Psychol 1988 (44):756-759
19 Metz CE: Basic principles of ROC analysis. Semin Nucl Med 1978 (8):283-298
20 Erdreich LS and Lee ET: Use of Relative Operating Characteristic analysis in epidemiology. Am J Epidemiol 1981 (114):649-662
21 Mari JJ and Williams P: A comparison of the validity of two psychiatric screening questionnaires (GHQ-12 and SRQ-20) in Brazil using Relative Operating Characteristics (ROC) analysis. Psychol Med 1981 (15):651-659
22 Swets JA: Indices of discrimination or diagnostic accuracy: their ROCS and implied models. Psychol Bull 1986 (99):100-117
23 Murphy JM, Berwick DM, Weinstein MC, Borus JF, Budman SH and Klerman GL: Performance of screening and diagnostic tests. Application of Receiver Operating Characteristic analysis. Arch Gen Psychiatry 1987 (44):550-555
24 Feinstein AR: Diagnostic and spectral markers. In: Feinstein AR (ed) Clinical Epidemiology: The Architecture of Clinical Research. WB Saunders Co, Philadelphia 1985 pp 597-631
25 Razavi D, Delvaux N, Farvacques C and Robaye E: The screening of adjustment disorders and major depressive disorders in hospitalized cancer patients (submitted for publication)
26 Hoopwood P, Howell A and Maguire P: Psychiatric morbidity in patients with advanced cancer of the breast. II. Prevalence measured by two self-rating questionnaires (submitted for publication)
28 Endicott J: Measurement of depression in patients with cancer. Cancer Suppl 1984 (53):2243-2250

Quality of Life Assessment in Cancer Clinical Trials

Neil K. Aaronson

Department of Psychosocial Research, The Netherlands Cancer Institute, Plesmanlaan 121, 1066 CX Amsterdam, The Netherlands

Over the past decade there has been an increasing interest in broadening the scope of evaluation parameters used in clinical research in oncology beyond the traditional indicators of therapeutic success such as prolonged survival, retardation of the disease process and control of major physical symptoms. It has been argued that assessment of the efficacy of cancer therapies requires greater attention to the impact of treatment on the functional, psychological and social health of the individual. While a range of terms have been applied to this expanded evaluation focus, it is frequently subsumed under the heading of "quality of life" research.

While the term "quality of life" as it has been applied in the health care field is of relatively recent vintage (e.g., it was introduced as a key word in medical literature databases only in 1975), one can trace its modern conceptual basis to the 1947 World Health Organisation definition of health as "a state of complete physical, mental and social well-being, and not merely the absence of disease and infirmity" [1]. Several years later, Karnofsky and Burchenal [2] signalled the introduction of psychosocial or quality-of-life variables in clinical cancer research in their seminal article on the evaluation of new chemotherapeutic agents. In that article, they identified four sets of criteria necessary for such evaluations: (a) subjective improvement; (b) objective improvement; (c) performance status; and (d) length of remission and prolongation of life. In contemporary terms, their "subjective improvement" criterion can be seen as reflecting basic quality-of-life considerations:

> "The patient's subjective improvement is measured or described in terms of improvement in his mood and attitude, his general feelings of well-being, his activity, appetite, and the alleviation of distressing symptoms, such as pain, weakness and dyspnoea." [2: pp 193-194].

The growing interest in quality-of-life considerations in oncology can be traced to a number of sources. Perhaps most importantly, it reflects the plateau that has been reached in the search for effective forms of treatment. While we have certainly witnessed significant therapeutic advances, for the major tumours (breast, lung, gastrointestinal) progress has been quite modest when viewed in terms of improved survival rates [3,4]. Much current clinical research is directed toward developing less toxic or less mutilating forms of treatment, rather than toward increasing survival rates *per se*. Where improved survival is a primary research objective, the intensive treatments employed often carry with them a high risk of treatment-related morbidity and mortality. The introduction of quality-of-life evaluations is a logical outgrowth of such a research focus.

The patients' rights movement in general, and particulary the demands of formal informed consent procedures, is also a relevant factor. Patients are demanding more information about the relative risks and benefits of alternative treatments. While clinicians may attend primarily to disease-oriented outcomes (e.g., tumour response), patients may be concerned equally with the impact of therapies on their daily lives. Quality-of-life data provide one approach to translating medical

outcomes into terms that are more recognisable and meaningful to the patient and his family.
Finally, the large body of descriptive literature in psychosocial oncology has underscored the value of incorporating the patient's perspective in our research, and of approaching cancer as an illness (a social phenomenon) as well as a disease process. A study by Coates and his colleagues [5] of patients undergoing chemotherapy illustrates this point rather nicely. In this study, patients were asked to rate the relative importance of a large set of possible physical and nonphysical side effects of their treatment. As would be expected, those side effects cited most frequently include such common physical symptoms as nausea, vomiting, fatigue and alopecia. Yet, also included among the most frequently noted side effects were anxiety, depression, sleep disturbance and the negative impact of the treatment on family, work and social activities. Such "quality-of-life toxicities" are not addressed by the classical rating systems employed in oncological research.

Quality-of-Life Research Applications

As illustrated briefly above, at the most basic level quality-of-life assessments can aid in the monitoring of the effect of standard therapies on the daily lives of patients, often with an eye toward improving the ways in which treatments are delivered (e.g., reducing the number of drugs administered or the overall duration of exposure).
When carried out on a sufficiently large scale, descriptive quality-of-life studies can help to establish norms regarding both the short-term and long-term psychosocial adjustment of patients (e.g., the prevalence of psychological depression among surgically-treated breast cancer patients during the first postoperative year; the prevalence of sexual dysfunction among testicular cancer survivors 5 years after treatment). In turn, such norms can be used in screening programmes aimed at identifying high-risk groups or individuals who might benefit most from targeted psychosocial interventions. For example, Maguire and his colleagues [6] developed a screening programme to identify candidates for formal psychological counselling following mastectomy. Such counselling would be far too costly if provided to all post-mastectomy patients. By establishing appropriate screening procedures, funds for supportive services could be allocated more efficiently.
Perhaps the most promising direction for quality-of-life research is in the realm of phase III clinical trials. The overriding objective in such studies is to identify the best therapeutic approach among competing treatments. Quality-of-life parameters can be viewed as a means of redefining and refining what we mean by "best." Frequently, quality-of-life substudies are used to confirm empirically certain clinical impressions regarding the psychosocial benefits of one clinical approach over another. This is the case, for example, in randomised studies comparing the psychosocial sequelae of breast-conserving therapy versus mastectomy. In general, these studies have supported the assumption that the less mutiliating forms of surgery yield significant psychosocial gains (e.g., better body image, fewer sexual problems) [7-9].
Conversely, the results of clinical trial based quality-of-life investigations can sometimes challenge widely held beliefs. For example, it has often been argued that breast-conserving therapy, while holding certain psychosocial advantages over mastectomy, nevertheless increases a woman's fear of disease recurrence. Yet, empirical investigations have not generally lent support to this contention [7-9]. Similarly, in a recent controlled trial in advanced breast cancer [10], the hypothesis that an intermittent chemotherapy schedule would improve patients' quality of life as compared with a continuous regimen, was not confirmed. To the contrary, continuous therapy resulted in significant improvements in quality of life as compared with the interrupted schedule. Other "counter-intuitive" quality-of-life findings have been reported in studies comparing a "wait-and-see" approach with adjuvant chemotherapy in operable breast cancer [11], and limb-sparing procedures versus amputation in soft-tissue sarcoma [12].

Barriers to the Introduction of Quality-of-Life Assessment in Cancer Clinical Trials

Despite their demonstrated utility, inclusion of quality-of-life parameters in clinical trials remains the exception rather than the rule. In a review of cancer clinical trials undertaken between 1956 and 1976, Bardelli and Saracci [13] reported that fewer than 5% of published studies employed quality-of-life outcomes. In a more recent literature review encompassing the period 1981-1986, only 3 of 99 published studies of surgical trials included quality-of-life evaluations [14].

Much of the hesitancy in adopting psychosocial research strategies in clinical trials would appear to derive from a basic lack of familiarity of the clinical and social science research communities with one another. On the one hand, clinical researchers are typically untrained in, and perhaps also a bit distrustful of, social science research methodologies. On the other hand, social scientists often fail to familiarise themselves sufficiently with the substantive research questions of interest to clinicians, and frequently exhibit a lack of sensitivity to the practical constraints operating within clinical trial settings.

A particularly thorny problem is the lack of consensus on how quality of life should be measured. The physician interested in assessing the psychosocial impact of both routine medical care and experimental treatments is confronted with a confusing array of choices. At one end of the spectrum are extensive and time-consuming interview protocols that exceed the practical limits present in most clinical settings. At the other end are more concise patient self-report questionnaires which, while representing a less cumbersome approach to data collection, often leave unanswered the critical questions of instrument reliability and validity.

Similarly, psychosocial research designs are often viewed by those responsible for conducting clinical trials as overly burdensome both to themselves and to their patients. Such perceived burden may result, in part, from a basic lack of familiarity with the nature and intent of the psychosocial assessments. It also reflects, however, inexperience on the part of social scientists with the realities of clinical practice. Data collection schemes often call for frequent application of questionnaires during the rush of outpatient clinics. While such procedures can, in theory, yield a rich data base, they do not attend sufficiently to the practical constraints involved.

The remainder of this chapter will be devoted to a discussion of a range of conceptual, methodological and practical issues surrounding the introduction of quality-of-life assessments in cancer clinical trials. The four broad areas to be addressed include: (a) the appropriate source of quality-of-life data; (b) defining and operationalising health-related quality of life; (c) factors to consider in selecting or developing quality-of-life measures; and (d) quality-of-life research design and implementation.

Who Should Measure Quality of Life?

The quality of life of patients can be assessed by a health care provider, by the patient him or herself, or by someone close to the patient such as a partner or other family member. Historically, it has most often been the physician who has provided such assessments, albeit in a limited way. In most clinical trials in oncology clinicians are asked to assess both the performance status of their patients (using either the 11-step Karnofksy scale [2] or alternative rating systems [15]), as well as the clinical toxicities associated with the treatment. More recently, physician-based rating systems have been developed to address a broader set of quality-of-life dimensions, including psychological and social well-being [16].

The principal advantages associated with such clinician-based observation techniques are of a practical nature. Typically, it requires much less time and effort to complete a rating form oneself than it does to arrange for patients to be interviewed or to be assisted in filling out a questionnaire. Yet, the available evidence suggests that methodological limitations associated with these scales may outweigh their practical advantages. Several studies have documented low levels of inter-observer reliability and, perhaps more importantly, low levels of agreement between ratings provided by physicians and those of patients themselves [17-19]. There is some evidence indicating that the reliability of clinician-based rating scales can be improved significantly by introducing standardised instructions and by providing training in their use [20,21]. Additionally, data suggest that nurses and other ancillary health care personnel may provide more reliable ratings than do physicians [22].

In the light of these considerations, it is not surprising that most workers in the field lobby for direct questioning of patients about the impact of disease and treatment on their daily lives. This is clearly desirable when one is interested in assessing such subjective experiences as pain, fatigue or psychological distress. Yet, even in the case of more readily observable symptoms (e.g., alopecia among chemotherapy patients), patient feedback may provide important insights into their meaning and impact on daily living.

Feedback provided by a family member can yield useful supplementary information regarding the patient's quality of life. In studies involving children, the parents may serve as the primary source of such data. Yet, even in the case of the adult patient, the partner may provide a unique perspective regarding such issues as mood state, functional capacity and level of sexual interest. Nevertheless, due to both ethical and logistical considerations, use of "significant others" to inform us about the quality of life of trial patients should probably be restricted to selective cases.

A Quality-of-Life Taxonomy

Just as cancer is a collective noun for some 100 forms of disease [4], so is quality of life a collective term summarising a set of related, interacting dimensions. Attempts to establish boundaries around the term have proven difficult. As Feinstein [23] puts it: "The idea has become a kind of umbrella under which are placed many different indexes dealing with whatever the user wants to focus on."

One way of circumventing the problem of concept definition is to remain at a global level, leaving the quality-of-life term essentially undefined. For example, Gough and his coworkers [24] suggest that one need only field a single question to evaluate cancer patients' quality of life: "How would you rate your quality of life today?" They support their position by demonstrating a relatively strong correlation between scores on this single item and scores derived from more elaborate assessment batteries. Unfortunately, such statistical evidence begs the issue of utility. While it may be useful to have a summary quality-of-life score for certain tasks (e.g., for calculating quality-adjusted life years), more specific information is required in order to understand such global ratings. How are we to interpret a patient reporting a low quality of life? Does it imply limitations in functional capacity, intolerable symptoms levels, depression, social isolation, or a combination of such factors?

An approach that has been applied frequently in population-based social indicators research is to define quality of life in terms of a subjective judgement of the degree to which happiness, satisfaction or a sense of well-being has been attained. Aside from the tautological problem inherent in such a definition (i.e., Why do I have a good quality of life? Because I am happy. Why am I happy? Because I have a good quality of life), it is questionable whether such broad issues should be the focus in health-related quality-of-life research. Adoption of such an approach would imply that the health care system has responsibility for attaining such societal goals as happiness and life satisfaction. This would seem to overstep the mandate that most societies impose on their health care professionals.

A more modest and realistic approach is to limit our focus to those issues where it can be reasonably expected that the health care system can have a direct impact [25]. Within such a health-related framework, there appears to be a growing consensus that quality of life is a multidimensional construct composed minimally of the following four domains: (a) functional status; (b) disease-related and treatment-related symptoms; (c) psychological functioning; and (d) social functioning [26]. While a comprehensive discussion of each of these domains is beyond the scope of this paper, a number of central issues related to their measurement bear mentioning.

Functional Status

Functional status refers to the ability to perform a range of activities that are normal for most people (often age-adjusted). Four categories of functioning measured most commonly include: (a) self-care (e.g., feeding, dressing, bathing and using the toilet); (b) mobility (i.e., the ability to move about indoors and outdoors); (c) physical activities (e.g., walking, climbing stairs); and (d) role actitivies (i.e., social roles associated with work and family) [27].

A large number of patient self-report measures are available to assess functional status [28]. However, many of these measures have been developed for use among patient populations with very limited functional capacities (e.g., patients with severe, debilitating arthritis), and thus are probably too crude to be used among cancer populations.

A second issue to be considered in selecting among available measures is the extent to which they take level of effort into consideration. Two individuals may be able to carry out the same level of activity (e.g., walking stairs), but with very different degrees of effort.

Disease-Related and Treatment-Related Symptoms

Each form of cancer has its own natural history and characteristic behaviour. Similarly, each therapeutic intervention or combination of interventions carries with it specific toxcities. Nevertheless, a core set of physical symptoms can be identified which are reported commonly by cancer patients, either as a result of the disease or of the treatment. These include fatigue and malaise, dyspnoea, pain, weight loss, appetite loss, nausea and vomiting, alopecia and sleep disturbance.

Notation of disease symptoms and treatment side effects is typically a mandatory part of clinical trials. It is important to stress that, due to the subjective nature of many of these symptoms, direct and standardised questioning of patients is essential. Each symptom can be assessed in a variety of ways, ranging from a simple dichotomous variable representing its presence or absence, to more refined measures of frequency, severity of occurrence and duration. In general, the use of a frequency or severity rating scale can be recommended as it can capture gradations in symptom experience which may not be noted with a cruder measure of presence/absence.

Psychological Functioning

Despite the relatively large number of studies that have investigated the psychological status of cancer patients, the prevalence of psychiatric disability among this population remains unclear. For example, the prevalence rate for depression reported in various studies ranges from less than 5% [29] to approximately 50% [30]. Massie and Holland [31] note that the highest rates of depression among cancer patients are found in studies that rely on clinicians' judgements, and that involve patients with more advanced disease and more severe illness levels. In fact, the variability in estimates can be accounted for by a number of factors, including: (a) heterogeneity of patient samples in terms of stage of disease, time since diagnosis, and nature and stage of treatment; (b) lack of agreement on conceptualisation of primary psychiatric concepts; (c) diversity of assessment techniques employed; and (d) methodological problems such as small sample sizes, biased sample selection, and ambiguous time frames for assessing symptomatology.

Many of the studies of the psychological status of cancer patients cannot be interpreted in terms of pathological states or diagnosable mental disorder. Rather, they indicate a more generalised, nonspecific form of distress reflecting the impact of the diagnosis of cancer, reaction to the progression of the disease, or the side effects of treatment [32,33].

A variety of measures are available for assessing psychological morbidity, ranging from extensive psychiatric interviews to multidimensional self-report symptom checklists to unidimensional scales. However, within the context of clinical trials, the choice of measures may be quite restricted. Clearly, lengthy, omnibus instruments designed to assess psychological status in a comprehensive sense cannot be employed for reasons of practicality. Yet, even within the narrower range of unidimensional measures, certain cautions should be exercised. Of particular importance is to avoid the use of instruments that rely heavily on physical symptoms (e.g., tiredness, decreased sexual drive, appetite loss) to establish the presence of emotional problems. Among cancer patients, it may be difficult to determine if such symptoms are somatic manifestations of psychological disturbance or are related directly to the disease and its treatment [34].

Social Functioning

Disruption of normal social activities and relationships may be experienced by cancer patients at various stages in the disease trajectory. Functional problems due to pain or fatigue, as well as the demands of treatment regimens, may place serious limitations and strains on the ability to maintain social contacts [35].

Psychological reactions of the cancer patient may also lead to restricted social contacts. Fear of being a burden to others, feelings of embarrassment about symptoms or disability and fear of rejection may lead to avoidance of social situations and a hesitancy in asking for support [35,36].

Family and friends may reduce their level of contact with the cancer patient, or alter their normal patterns of communication to "protect" the patient from the stresses associated with everyday life. Similarly, they may avoid talking about the disease and its treatment out of feelings of awkwardness or fear of inadequacy [37,38]. In extreme cases, lack of understanding of the nature of cancer may result in avoidance of contact altogether (e.g., out of fear of contagion).

Although the negative consequences of cancer for the social health of the individual are most often discussed, it should be emphasised that the crisis of cancer can also lead to a strengthening and enrichment of social relationships [39]. In fact, a number of studies indicate that patients often perceive the degree of support that they receive from their social network as more than adequate [40,41].

Assessment of social functioning can be affected by an underreporting bias. Patients may be hesitant to report problems in their social sphere if questions are phrased in terms that imply criticism of family members and friends. By focussing on the behavioural aspects of interpersonal relationships (e.g., the ability to maintain normal social contacts), rather than on their affective dimensions (e.g., feelings of love and support), such bias may be minimised. In order to capture the full range of social health effects, measures should be chosen that also allow for reporting of the positive changes in the patient's social environment resulting from the cancer experience.

Additional Quality-of-Life Dimensions

Beyond this core set of quality-of-life domains there are a number of additional issues that may be of interest when studying specific groups of patients. Thus, for example, body image may be relevant in studies of patients treated for breast cancer, head-and-neck tumours and other forms of cancer that often involve mutilating treatment. Sexual functioning may be at issue for breast, gynaecological and male genito-urinary tract cancers. Cognitive functioning may be of particular concern in studies of childhood cancer or studies of adults with brain tumours. Ultimately, the combination of quality-of-life domains assessed in a given study is a function of the patient population under consideration, the nature of the applied treatments and the specific research questions at hand.

Finally, because quality of life is undoubtedly more than the sum of its component parts, it may be useful to include a global assessment as a supplement, rather than as an alternative, to more specific measures. Such global measures may be useful in interpreting the relative importance of the more specific quality-of-life domains measured, and can be used as summary measures in analyses involving qualitative adjustment of survival data.

Issues in Selecting or Developing Quality-of-Life Measures

Although a relatively large number of instruments are available to measure health-related quality of life, there is a tendency in this field of research to try out new assessment approaches rather than to draw upon existing resources. Dependent on the specificity of the research question at hand, the development of a new instrument may well be warranted. Frequently, however, the decision to "reinvent the wheel" appears to reflect the system of rewards operating in the social sciences, rather than a legitimate gap in the available resource pool. Just as original research carries with it more professional payoff than efforts at synthesising exisiting knowledge, instrument development is often more highly valued than instrument adaptation. One cannot help feeling that, if more effort were invested in the admittedly cumbersome task of reviewing the available literature, the perceived need for undertaking the even more difficult task of instrument development would diminish.

In fact, there are a number of excellent sources that provide an overview of extant instruments in the quality of life and health status measurement fields [cf. 42-47]. In the current discussion, we will focus on some of the more generic issues involved in selecting among available measures, with instrument development being consigned to a parenthetical position. In practice, of course, the relevant issues are much the same in both situations.

Broad Versus Narrow Topic Coverage

As noted earlier, quality of life is most often approached as a multifaceted concept. Thus, quality-of-life investigations tend to be characterised by the use of either a battery of measures, or a single instrument that incorporates a number of discrete subscales. However, given the practical constraints surrounding the collection of patient self-report data (i.e., the need to limit the total number of questions asked and the time demanded of patients), the investigator is typically confronted with a choice of degrees between breadth and depth of coverage. Some studies attempt to capture the complexity of the quality-of-life construct by assessing the widest possible range of psychosocial issues. Other investigations are more circumscribed in their scope, offering instead a greater depth of inquiry per topic.

While the balance to be struck between breadth and depth of inquiry depends on the nature of the research question at hand, Ware [48] suggests that routine assessment of a fairly broad, comprehensive set of psychosocial variables may often be most appropriate given our limited knowledge of the impact of chronic disease on everyday functioning. Similarly, the psychosocial trade-offs associated with alternative treatments are often poorly understood. At the same time, however, casting a wide assessment net does not justify an investigative "fishing expedition." Ultimately, decisions regarding the scope of measurement should be guided by our current level of knowledge of the psychosocial health status of the specific patient population of interest. In those cases where the available literature is scanty, broad coverage of issues may be most appropriate. In relatively well-studied areas, the pressing need may be for a more detailed and sophisticated exploration of a limited number of topics.

Interviews, Questionnaires or Diaries

Interviews represent an extremely flexible form of data collection in the social sciences. The principal advantages associated with interview techniques are that: (a) they can be applied to the broadest range of patients, including those who might otherwise have difficulty in completing a self-report questionnaire (e.g., the elderly, poorly educated or physically handicapped; (b) they facilitate sophisticated question branching; (c) they can minimise the problem of missing data by incorporating probes for clarification or amplification of patients' responses; and (d) they allow for the collection of additional observational or non-verbal information.

Offsetting these advantages is the fact that interviews require more commitment of staff time than is typically available in clinical settings. Particularly in multi-centre studies, it cannot be expected that sufficient resources will be available to permit interviews as the standard method of data collection. Where interviews are feasible, careful training and quality control is needed to minimise potential bias and errors due to inexperienced (or sometimes overexperienced) interviewers.

Self-administered questionnaires, while often sacrificing the richness of detail obtained via interviews, represent a practical, efficient and relatively inexpensive form of data collection. Particularly in clinical trials or prospective studies, written questionnaires can ease the task of collecting information over time. There is also evidence to suggest that some patients may prefer to respond to a written questionnaire rather than to an interviewer, particularly if the topics covered are of a sensitive nature [49].

Although the majority of available quality-of-life measures are designed to be self-administered, they can usually be easily adapted for interviewer administration. The reverse, however, is seldom the case. Measures originally designed as interviews will often contain question probes and skip patterns that would be confusing if used in a self-administered form.

Patient diaries are particularly useful if one is interested in frequent (e.g., daily) assessment of changes in symptom experience. For example, the British Medical Research Council has developed a diary card for use among patients receiving chemotherapy or radiotherapy which includes ratings of nausea and vomiting, activity level, mood state, anxiety and overall health [50]. The major limitation of diaries is that, due to the frequency of administration, the number of questions asked must remain quite limited. Further, patient compliance can be a significant problem that may remain undetected if patients complete the diary retrospectively (e.g., for an entire week). This, of course, would defeat the purpose of the diary approach.

Level of Data (Dis)Aggregation

An important issue to consider in choosing a quality-of-life measure is the degree of flexibility offered in terms of aggregating or disaggregating the data. The availability of procedures to aggregate individual items into a more discrete number of scales or indexes carries with it a number of psychometric advantages. Summative ratings can: (a) increase the variability of scores, an important requisite for detecting changes in health status over time and differences among patient groups; (b) increase score reliability by pooling information that items have in common; (c) increase score validity, if items are selected carefully to provide a representative sample of information; and (d) reduce missing data problems by providing the option, if responses to individual questions are missing, of estimating scores based on the remaining questions comprising the scale.

Most multidimensional quality-of-life measures permit some degree of data aggregation. If there is interest in combining quality-of-life outcomes with survival data (e.g., to estimate "quality-adjusted life years"), then one should look for an instrument that also yields a single, overall score. In general, however, measures that offer only such a global score, without the possibility of disaggregation, are not recommended due to the loss of information involved.

Time Frame of the Questions

Health-related quality-of-life measures employ a variety of question time frames. Patients may be asked to report on their experience of a given day, during the previous week, during the previous month, or even over a longer time period. Not infrequently, the time frame of the questions is left undefined.

In measuring psychosocial parameters in cancer clinical trials we may be interested in both the short-term and long-term effects of the disease and of the treatment. Particularly in assessing acute treatment effects, use of a short question time frame may be quite important. For example, during chemotherapy, two time periods can typically be distinguished: a period during which the immediate, acute effects of the drug are experienced (e.g., nausea and vomiting, fatigue); and a rest period during which the patient recovers from these immediate effects. In such situations, if the time frame of the questions is too long, or is left undefined, the patient may be confused as to which period he or she should report - the treatment period, the rest period, or perhaps both [51].

Even in the case of long-term effects, the use of a relatively short question time frame (e.g., one week) can be recommended. This will minimise problems associated with memory loss, and will avoid confounding specific symptom experience with a more generalised tendency to complain. This latter point was illustrated in a study by Huisman and his colleagues [52] in which subjects were asked to complete a symptom checklist, as well as several personality trait measures designed to assess a more general tendency to complain in either psychological or physical terms. They found that, as the time frame of the symptom checklist was lengthened, its correlation with the personality trait measures increased. With a 1-month time frame it was virtually impossible to distinguish between specific symptom experience and the more generalised personality trait. The authors concluded that one week is the maximum time frame that can be recommended to avoid such problems.

A related issue concerns the use of items that ask patients to evaluate their current condition in relation to how they "usually" or "normally" feel. While such questions may be appropriate when asked of healthy individuals, they can be quite confusing for patients with a chronic disease such as cancer. Patients may not know if they should compare their current situation with their pre-illness state, with their condition prior to receiving treatment, or with their average condition since being under treatment.

Response Scales

There are two principal methods for coding and quantifying responses to questionnaire or interview items: category ratings and linear analogue scales. Category ratings can take the form of either a simple dichotomous response (e.g., "yes" or "no"; "true" or "false") or a Likert scale (e.g., "never", "sometimes", "frequently", "always"). Dichotomous choices, because of their simplicity, facilitate the fielding of a large number of questions in a relatively short time period. However, they sacrifice the degrees of shading offered by Likert scales that may be important for detecting more subtle differences between individuals or within individuals over time.

Linear analogue scales are typically composed of a 10-centimeter line with descriptive anchors at each end (e.g., "no pain" and "the worst pain that I can imagine"). The patient is asked to mark the point on the line that most closely corresponds to his or her experience, and the distance from the anchor points is subsequently measured.

Linear analogue scales are purported to be highly sensitive to small changes in symptom levels [53]. Yet, a recent head-to-head comparison of the linear analogue and Likert approaches failed to detect any differences in scale sensitivity [54]. It is also argued that linear analogue scales more closely approximate true interval level measures than do their Likert counterparts; a feature that facilitates the use of a wider range of robust statistical techniques. However, practical limitations may outweigh these more formal considerations. While a number of investigators report successful use of linear analogue methods [55,56], others argue that the level of abstraction required by the technique is too great for many patients [50,57]. Additionally, preparing such data for computer entry (i.e., physically measuring the distance between each response and the scale anchor) can become quite cumbersome, particularly in larger, multicentre clinical trials. Thus, all things being considered, it would appear that the practical advantages of the Likert approach favour its use over linear analogues.

Psychometric Properties

An important consideration in choosing among candidate quality-of-life measures is the extent to which psychometric standards of reliability, validity and sensitivity are met. Within the context of clinical trials, *reliability* is most often reported in terms of internal consistency estimates. While no hard and fast rules exist regarding minimal standards of internal consistency, Ware [49] suggests values above 0.90 if the instrument is to be used for individual comparisons, while more liberal standards (e.g., above 0.50) can be applied for group comparisons.

A second approach to reliability testing is the test-retest method, whereby scores obtained at two or more points in time are compared. This technique is appropriate when one expects that what is being measured will exhibit stability over time (e.g., personality traits). However, because in clinical trials we are most often interested in assessing changes in symptoms and behaviour (i.e., health states), this method may be of limited value. Finally, if quality-of-life estimates are based on observer ratings (e.g., clinician-based performance status scales), inter-rater reliability procedures are most appropriate.

While estimating scale reliability is a fairly straightforward statistical process, establishing scale *validity* can be an extremely time-consuming process. At the most basic level, careful examination of the form and content of questions can provide invaluable information regarding the face validity of a measure (e.g., Are the questions open to multiple interpretation? Do they cover adequately the full range of relevant topics?).

While examination of the face validity of scale items does not involve any formal statistical procedures, it represents one of the most important steps in the validation process. In order to maximise the face validity of quality-of-life measures, it is useful to include a range of individuals (e.g., physicians, social scientists, methodologists *and* patients) in the development process. The value of patient input was underscored in a recent study in which questionnaire items generated by aphasic patients were compared with those developed by rehabilitation clinicians [58]. The results indicated that clinicians seriously underestimated the patients' focus on social needs, and generated items that were much less specific and concrete than those of the patients themselves.

Criterion validity involves testing a scale against some other empirical standard. For example, a self-report measure of breathlessness could be compared with results obtained from a treadmill test or a lung function test. Unfortunately, in quality-of-life research it is often difficult to identify criterion measures that are themselves valid and reliable (e.g., for assessing psychological or social dysfunctioning).

Construct validity refers to a family of procedures that has as a common denominator the examination of the pattern of correlations within and between various scales. To establish construct validity one looks for evidence of convergence among indicators of the same or similar theoretical constructs, and of divergence between indicators of unrelated constructs. For example, one would expect scales (and the individual items comprising those scales) intended to assess anxiety and depression, to correlate more highly with one another than with another scale designed to measure fatigue. If this proved not to be the case, then the validity of these scales would be called into question. The multitrait-multimethod analysis techniques developed by Campbell and Fiske [59] offer a useful framework for examining the construct validity of measures.

The *sensitivity* of an instrument to either intra-individual change over time or inter-individual differences, is an essential consideration in clinical trial-based quality-of-life research. In comparative studies, the degree of sensitivity demanded of an instrument is inversely related to the expected effect size (i.e., the magnitude of change or differences in quality-of-life parameters that one is interested in detecting). Unfortunately, very few available quality-of-life measures provide sensitivity data. However, evidence of low scale score variability may signal problems with instrument sensitivity as well.

It should be emphasised that the psychometric properties of an instrument cannot be assumed to hold across different populations. A quality-of-life measure validated in the general population may perform poorly when used with chronic disease populations. Similarly, a measure that is well validated for a specific patient population (e.g., cardiovascular disease patients) will not necessarily perform adequately when used among cancer patients. Even when used in a population similar to that on which the original validation work was carried out, instrument performance may not measure up to expectations. For example, in a recent trial in metastatic lung cancer [57], the psychometric performance of the cancer-specific quality-of-life measure employed (the Functional Living Index - Cancer or FLIC) fell far short of what had been expected based on the original validation work. The authors suspected that differences in the sociodemographic characteristics and functional impairment levels of the study samples might have accounted for these disappointing results. This suggests the need for a period of pretesting before deciding whether a candidate quality-of-life measure is the best choice for a given clinical trial.

A related issue concerns the cross-cultural application of quality-of-life measures. The large majority of available measures have been developed and validated in English-speaking countries. Because these measures were not, in the first instance, developed with an eye toward international use, their content reflects the cultural norms and linguistic styles of their countries of origin. Indeed, the term "quality of life" itself is relatively culture-bound, and is difficult to translate adequately into varied languages.

In translating an instrument from one language to another it is important to ensure that the questions remain as close to their original conceputal meaning as possible. While complete cross-cultural equivalence may not be attainable, the use of standard "forward-backward" translation procedures can alleviate many of the basic language problems [60]. This involves translating an instrument from the original language into the second language ("forward") and then back again into the original language ("backward"). At least two individuals fluent in both languages should be involved in this process (one to carry out the forward translation, and one the translation backward). Typically, this is an iterative process requiring a number of rounds before equivalence is best approximated. Further refinements can be achieved during early field testing where patients can be asked to identify any questions that were difficult or confusing. The rigor required during this preparatory stage cannot be overemphasised. Without appropriate attention to detail, cross-cultural errors may only be detected during data analysis, as one searches for explanations for poor scale performance.

Generic Versus Disease-Specific Measures

Quality-of-life measures can be organised along a continuum reflecting their intended spectrum of application: (a) *ad hoc*, study-specific measures; (b) instruments designed for a specific disease population (e.g., for primary breast cancer patients); (c) instruments with a broader disease orientation (e.g., for use with cancer populations in general); and (d) generic instruments designed for use across a wide range of chronic disease populations.

Unfortunately, it is the *ad hoc* approach that has, to date, dominated quality-of-life research within the clinical trial context. The obvious difficulty with this approach is that it does not allow for comparison of results across studies. Additionally, such study-specific measures are seldom submitted to rigorous psychometric testing.

Instruments designed for a specific patient population overcome, to a limited degree, the problems inherent in the *ad hoc* approach. Yet, primary reliance on this assessment strategy would still necessitate the generation of a large number of measures to cover the spectrum of patient populations of potential interest.

Recent efforts have been mounted to design a more generic class of quality-of-life measures intended for use with a broader range of related patient populations. Specific to oncology, these include the Functional Living Index - Cancer [61], the Quality of Life Index [62], the questionnaire developed by Selby and his colleagues [63] and the EORTC Core Quality of Life Questionnaire [64]. None of these measures has yet to undergo sufficient field testing to justify a recommendation for general use. Nevertheless, the measurement strategy which they incorporate holds the promise of reconciling the need for a sufficient degree of generalisability to permit cross-study comparisons with the need for targeted assessment of psychosocial problems specific to cancer patient populations.

Finally, the class of instruments that is most generic in nature offers a broad coverage of important psychosocial domains, and facilitates a step-wise process of instrument development, validation and revalidation with a range of chronic disease populations. It is no accident that reports of the psychometric performance of such generic measures as the Sickness Impact Profile [65], the Nottingham Health Profile [66], the Quality of Well-Being Scale [67] and the RAND Health Insurance Experiment measures [68] have appeared regularly in the research literature.

However, many of these generic measures are quite lengthy, which can present serious problems when used with seriously ill patients, or when the research design calls for repeated applications over time. An instrument developed recently at the RAND Corporation - The MOS Short-Form General Health Survey [69] - offers comprehensiveness and psychometric robustness, while remaining short enough (i.e., 20 items) for use in clinical trial settings.

A further limitation of such generic measures is that they may not address adequately certain issues of particular relevance in evaluating the effect of a given disease or treatment on quality of life (e.g., specific disease symptoms or treatment side effects; specific psychosocial issues such as sexuality and body image). This problem can be remedied by including supplementary items or scales that cover such topics in some detail.

Quality-of-Life Research Design and Implementation

Measurement issues are clearly of paramount importance in quality-of-life research in oncology. Yet, our experience within the EORTC has taught us that research design and implementation problems are often of equal importance. One cannot help suspecting that the paucity of published reports of clinical trial-based quality-of-life research reflects not only a hesitancy to undertake such studies in the first place, but also a failure to generate sufficient data from those studies that have been initiated.

This raises the issues of practicality, or what Feinstein [70] terms "sensibility", surrounding quality-of-life-research efforts. While there are many design issues relevant to the successful implementation of quality-of-life studies, two that deserve particular attention are the frequency and timing of data collection and the problem of patient accrual and differential loss to follow-up.

The Burden Associated with Quality-of-Life Data Collection

The question of how frequently, and at what points in time, the quality of life of trial patients should be assessed, is related closely to the issues of patient, staff and institutional burden. While tolerance for answering questions is related to a number of factors (e.g., age and education), among chronic disease populations the health condition of the patients may be a determing factor. Lengthy interviews or questionnaires may be quite taxing, particularly for advanced-disease patients and for patients undergoing intensive treatment. In longitudinal studies, the amount of effort demanded of patients should be evaluated not only in relation to their current health status, but also against expected changes (often deterioration) in health status over the course of the study.

Clinicians often tend to overestimate the burden associated with quality-of-life investigations. In practice, most patients seem to welcome the opportunity to talk about their illness and treatment experience [71]. In fact, it is sometimes difficult to carry out such data collection efficiently due to the patients' desire to expand on the topics being addressed. Nevertheless, it remains the responsibility of the investigator to keep the data collection procedures within reasonable limits, and to be sensitive to individual differences in tolerance for answering questions.

It is difficult to provide specific guidelines regarding the optimal frequency of quality-of-life data collection in clinical trials. In trials where there is primary interest in the short-term, acute effects of treatment, relatively frequent questionnaire administration (e.g., once per treatment cycle) may be appropriate, assuming that the total length of treatment is relatively short. In trials involving lengthier treatments, or where the focus is on long-term effects, it is common to gradually lengthen the period between questionnaire administrations. For example, in EORTC-based quality-of-life studies, the data collection scheme for long-term trials calls typically for questionnaires once monthly during the first several months, once every 3 months through the first year, and every 6 months thereafter.

In addition to frequency of administration, the timing of questionnaires can be of critical importance, particularly if one is interested in capturing acute treatment effects. For example, delay in distributing questionnaires intended to be completed by patients at the end of a cycle of chemotherapy may result in serious underreporting of symptoms (i.e., the patient may fill in the questionnaire during a rest period, where symptom experience is diminished). During long-term patient follow up, the precision with which questionnaires are distributed can often be relaxed, with approximate target dates sufficing. In all cases, it can be recommended that the data collection be planned around regularly scheduled medical visits. It is the rare hospital administrator (or patient, for that matter) who would accept additional clinic appointments only for the purpose of such data collection.

At a second level, one needs to be concerned with the level of staff burden associated with quality-of-life assessments. If it is expected that medical or nursing staff are to carry out the quality-of-life data collection, then the procedures should reflect an appreciation of the time constraints operating the typical clinical setting. Failure to do so will only lead to staff resentment and, ultimately, to unacceptable levels of missing data.

Finally, the level of institutional burden should be considered in planning a quality-of-life study. Most hospitals, even those with a strong tradition in clinical research, will not have the infrastructure necessary to carry out extensive psychosocial investigations. Such practical issues as the scheduling of interviews or questionnaire administrations around routine clinic appointments, the setting up of patient tracking or follow-up procedures and the merging of psychosocial and medical databases, need to be carefully worked out. Special consideration should be given to the statistical expertise available for such projects. It should not be assumed that biostatisticians who routinely handle the clinical data from a trial will have the background necessary for analysing psychosocial data. Conversely, statisicians well-versed in social science methdology will often be unfamiliar with the analytic procedures required for working with clinical outcomes (e.g., for generating quality-of-life-adjusted survival analyses).

Patient Accrual and Differential Loss to Follow Up

At each stage of the clinical trial process, bias can be introduced that may compromise the representativeness of the study sample and, in extreme cases, may render the quality-of-life results impossible to interpret.

The first source of bias can be found at the institutional level. In many large-scale, multicentre clinical trials, quality-of-life assessment is an optional component of the research design. Often, the institutions that are willing to undertake quality-of-life investigations have academic affiliations or can otherwise be regarded as centres of "research excellence". Such institutions may have patient populations that are quite different from the more typical regional hospital. Thus, one runs the risk of accruing patients onto quality-of-life studies who are not representative of the sample of patients entered into the medical trial as a whole, let alone of the larger patient population of interest.

One way of eliminating this form of bias is to integrate quality-of-life studies as a mandatory component of trials. It is questionable, however, whether trial coordinators would be willing to risk the loss of potential institutional participation because of an unwillingness or inability of certain centres to collect psychosocial data. More realisitic measures that can be taken to maximise participation in quality-of-life studies include: (a) assuring that the purpose and value of collecting quality-of-life data are clearly stated in study protocols; (b) employing simple quality-of-life study designs that make minimal demands on medical staff; and (c) where feasible and apppropriate, offering additional (financial) incentives for participation in such studies.

In principle, once a centre has agreed to collect quality-of-life information, it is expected that all trial patients from that centre will be approached to take part in the study. In practice, however, this is often not the case. More typically, one finds that only a percentage of the trial patients are included in the quality-of-life study. When queried, physicians will most often attribute this to administrative mistakes, hectic outpatient clinics and other such external factors. If this were always the case, there would be little reason for concern. Yet, one cannot help suspecting that some patients are excluded from quality-of-life investigations for more substantive reasons (e.g., the physician feels that the patient is too upset, or that the doctor-patient relationship would be affected adversely). If such systematic selection takes place, the representativeness of the quality-of-life sample would be further compromised.

Again, use of a realistic data collection scheme that minimises the disruption of normal clinic routine can eliminate many of the administrative problems surrounding quality-of-life data collection. Use of certain data management tools such as study calendars and flagging of patient charts can also facilitate smoother study administration. Exclusion of patients from study participation on *a priori* grounds is a more intransigent problem. While the evidence suggests that the vast majority of patients are willing to take part in quality-of-life studies, it is only through experience that the individual physician can be convinced of the relatively benign (and often beneficial) nature of patient participation in such research.

The final and most serious form of bias occurs when patients are lost to follow-up. Frequently, as patients become more ill and symptomatic, they will be incapable of completing a questionnaire or unwilling to do so. Yet, it is precisely at this point of disease progression that we are most interested in assessing changes in quality of life. It may be possible to lengthen the period that patients remain on-study by assuring that assistance is available for completing questionnaires, or that questionnaires can be administered in the form of a brief interview. Ultimately, of course, concern with the well-being of the patient must outweigh considerations surrounding the methodological integrity of a study.

Conclusions

There is currently a great deal of interest in assessing the quality of life of cancer patients. One of the more promising directions in this area of research is the incorporation of quality-of-life assessments into clinical trials. In order to maximise the likelihood that quality-of-life data will attain a legitimate place in the clinical research process, care must be taken in developing brief, well-designed instruments that meet rigorous scientific standards. At the same time, quality-of-life research designs must reflect an appreciation of the practical constraints operating in the typical clinical setting. Underlying these technical issues is the continuing need to refine our understanding of the relationship between disease as a biological process and illness as a social phenomenon. Ultimately, the goal is to develop evaluation models that achieve a sophisticated balance between qualitative and quantitative definitions of therapeutic success.

REFERENCES

1 World Health Organization: The constitution of the World Health Organization. WHO Chronicle 1947 (1):29

2 Karnofsky DA and Burchenal JH: Clinical evaluation of chemotherapeutic agents in cancer. In: MacLeod CM (ed) Evaluation of Chemotherapeutic Agents. Columbia University Press, New York 1949 pp 191-205

3 Bailar JC and Smith EM: Progress against cancer? NEJM 1986 (19):1226-1232

4 Cairns J: The treatment of disease and the war against cancer. Sci Am 1985 (253):31-39

5 Coates A, Abraham S, Kaye SB et al: On the receiving end: Patient perception of the side effects of cancer chemotherapy. Eur J Clin Oncol 1985 (19):203-208

6 Maguire P, Tait A, Brooke M et al: Effect of counseling on the psychiatric morbidity associated with mastectomy. Br Med J 1980 (281):1454-1455

7 de Haes JCJM, van Oostrom MA and Welvaart K: Quality of life after breast cancer surgery. J Surg Oncol 1985 (28):123-125

8 Kemeny MM, Wellisch DK and Schain WS: Psychosocial outcome in a randomized surgical trial for treatment of primary breast cancer. Cancer 1988 (62):1231-1237

9 Lasry JCM, Margolese RG, Poisson R et al: Depression and body image following mastectomy and lumpectomy. J Chron Dis 1987 (40):529-534

10 Coates A, Gebski V, Stat M et al: Improving the quality of life during chemotherapy for advanced breast cancer. NEJM 1987 (317):1490-1495

11 Gelber RD and Goldhirsch A: A new endpoint for the assessment of adjuvant therapy in postmenopausal women with operable breast cancer. J Clin Oncol 1986 (4):1772-1779

12 Sugarbaker Ph, Barofsky I, Rosenberg SA et al: Quality of life assessment of patients in extremity sarcoma clinical trials. Surgery 1982 (91):17-23

13 Bardelli D and Saracci R: Measuring the quality of life in cancer clinical trials: A sample survey of published trials. In: Armitage P (ed) Methods and Impact of Controlled Therapeutic Trials in Cancer, Part 1. International Union Against Cancer, Geneva 1978 pp 75-94

14 O'Young J and McPeek B: Quality of life variables in surgical trials. J Chron Dis 1987 (40):513-522

15 Zubrod CG, Scheiderman M, Frei E et al: Cancer - appraisal of methods for the study of chemotherapy of cancer in man: thiophosphoramide. J Chron Dis 1960 (11):7-33

16 Spitzer WO, Dobson AJ, Hall J, Chesterman E, Levi J, Shepherd R, Battista RN and Catchlove BR: Measuring the quality of life of cancer patients: A concise QL-index for use by physicians. J Chron Dis 1981 (34):585-597

17 Hutchinson TA, Boyd NF and Feinstein AR: Scientific problems in clinical scales as demonstrated by the Karnofsky index of performance status. J Chron Dis 1979 (32):661-666

18 Schag CC, Heinrich RL and Ganz PA: Karnofsky performance status revisited: Reliability, validity and guidelines. J Clin Oncol 1984 (2):187-193

19 Slevin ML, Plant H, Lynch D, Drinkwater J and Gregory WM: Who should measure quality of life, the doctor or the patient? Br JCancer 1988 (57):109-112

20 Grieco A and Long CJ: Investigations of the Karnofsky performance status as a measure of quality of life. Hlth Psych 1984 (3):129-142

21 Mor V, Laliberte L and Morris JN: The Karnofsky performance status scale: An examination of its reliability and validity in a research setting. Cancer 1984 (53):2002-2007

22 Yates JW, Chalmer B and McKegney FP: Evaluation of patients with advanced cancer using the Karnofksy performance status. Cancer 1980 (45):2220-2224

23 Feinstein AR: Clinimetric perspectives. J Chron Dis 1987 (40):635-640

24 Gough IR, Furnival CM, Schilder I et al: Assessment of the quality of life of patients with advanced cancer. Eur J CancerClin Oncol 1983 (19):1161-1165

25 Ware JE: Standards for validating health measures: Definition and content. J Chron Dis 1987 (40):473-480

26 de Haes JCJM and van Knippenberg FCE: The quality of life of cancer patients: A review of the literature. Soc Sci Med 1985 (20):809-817

27 Stewart AI, Ware JE, Brook RH and Davies-Avery A: Conceptualization and Measurment of Health for Adults in the Health Insurance Study Vol 2, Physical Health in Terms of Functioning. The Rand Corporation, R-1987/2-HEW, Santa Monica, CA 1978

28 Feinstein AR, Josephy BR and Wells CK: Scientific and clinical problems in indexes of functional disability. Ann Internal Med 1986 (105):413-420

29 Lansky SB, List MA, Herrman CA et al: Absence of major depressive disorders in female cancer patients. J Clin Oncol 1985 (3):1553-1560

30 Derogatis LR, Morrow GR, Fetting J et al: The prevalence of psychiatric disorders among cancer patients. JAMA 1983 (249):751-757

31 Massie MJ and Holland JC: Assessment and management of the cancer patient with depression. Adv Psychosom Med 1988 (18):1-12

32 Greer S and Silberfarb PM: Psychological concomitants of cancer: Current state of research. Psychol Med 1982 (12):563-573

33 Worden JW and Weisman AD: Preventive psychosocial intervention with newly diagnosed cancer patients. Gen Hosp Psychiatry 1984 (6):243-249

34 Endicott J: Measurement of depression in patients with cancer. Cancer 1984 (53):2243-2248

35 Bury M: Chronic illness as biographical disruption. Sociology Hlth Illness 1982 (41):167-182

36 Strauss HM and Glaser: Chronic Illness and the Quality of Life. Mosby, New York 1975

37 Peters-Golden H: Breast cancer: Varied perceptions of social support in the illness experience. Soc Sci Med 1982 (16):483-491

38 Wortman CB: Social support and the cancer patient: Conceptual and methodological issues. Cancer 1983 (53):2217-2384

39 Taylor SE, Falke RL, Shoptaw SJ and Lichtman RR: Social support, support groups and the cancer patient. J Consult Clin Psych 1986 (54):608-615

40 Dunkel-Schetter C: Social support and cancer. Findings based on patient interviews and their implications. J Social Issues 1984 (40):77-98

41 Lichtman RR and Taylor SE: Close relationships and the female cancer patient. In Andersen BL (ed) Women with Cancer: Psychological Perspectives. Springer-Verlag, New York 1986 pp 233-256

42 Wenger NK, Mattson ME, Furberg CD and Elinson J (ed) Assessment of Quality of Life in Clinical Trials of Cardiovascular Therapies. Le Jacq, New York 1984

43 McDowell I and Newell C: Measuring Health: A Guide to Rating Scales and Questionnaires. Oxford University Press, Oxford 1987

44 Adam J: Quality of Life and Cancer. World Health Organization Regional Office for Europe, Copenhagen 1986

45 Walker SR (ed) Quality of Life Assessment and Application. MTP Press Limited, The Hague 1988

46 Self P and Robertson B: Measurement of quality of life in patients with cancer. Cancer Surveys 1987 (6): 521-543

47 de Haes JCJM and Knippenberg FCE: Quality of life of cancer patients: Review of the literature. Soc Sci Med 1985 (20):809-817

48 Ware JE: Conceptualizing disease impact and treatment outcomes. Cancer 1984 (53):2216-2326

49 Ware JE: Methodological considerations in the selection of health status assessment procedures. In: Wenger NK, Mattson ME, Furberg CD and Elinson J (eds) Assessment of Quality of Life in Clinical Trials of Cardiovascular Therapies. Le Jacq, New York 1984 pp 87-112

50 Fayers PM and Jones SDR: Measuring and analyzing the quality of life in cancer clinical trials: A review. Statistics in Medicine 1983 (2):429-446

51 van Dam FSAM, Linssen CAG, and Couzijn AL: Evaluating 'quality of life' in cancer clinical trials. In Buyse M, Staquet M and Sylvester R (eds) Cancer Clinical Trials: Methods and Practice. Oxford University Press, London 1984 pp 26-43

52 Huisman SJ, van Dam FSAM, Aaronson NK and Hanewald G: On measuring complaints of cancer patients: Some remarks on the time span of the question. In Aaronson NK, Beckmann J, Bernheim J and Zittoun R (eds) The Quality of Life of Cancer Patients. Raven Press, New York 1987 pp 101-109

53 Huskisson EC, Jones J and Scott PJ: Applications of visual analogue scales to the measurement of functional capacity. Rheum Rehabil 1976 (15):185-187.

54 Guyatt GH, Townsend M, Berman L and Keller JL: A comparison of likert and visual analogue scales for measuring change in function. J Chron Dis 1987 (40):1129-1133

55 Priestman TJ and Baum M: Evaluation of quality of life in patients receiving treatment for advanced breast cancer. Lancet1976 (1):899-900

56 Padilla G, Presant C, Grant M, Metter G, Lipsett J and Heide F: Quality of life index for patients with cancer. Res Nurs Health1983 (6):117-126

57 Ganz PA, Haskell CM, Figlin RA, La Soto N and Siaus J: Estimating the quality of life in a clinical trial of patients with metastatic lung cancer using the Karnofsky performance status and the Functional Living Index-Cancer. Cancer 1988 (61):849-856

58 Lomas J, Pickard L and Mohide A: Patient versus clinician item generation for quality of life measures. Medical Care 1987 (25):764-769

59 Campbell D and Fiske DW: Convergent and discriminant validation by the multitrait-multimethod matrix. Psychol Bull 1959 (56):81-105

60 Sartorius N: Crosscultural Psychiatry. Springer-Verlag, Berlin 1979

61 Schipper H, Clinich J, McMurray A and Levitt M: Measuring the quality of life of cancer patients: The Functional Living Index - Cancer. J Clin Oncol 1984 (2):472-483

62 Padilla GV, Presant C, Grant MM, Metter G, Lipsett J and Heide F: Quality of life index for patients with cancer. Res Nurs Health 1983 (6):117-126

63 Selby PJ, Chapman JA, Etazadi-Amoli J, Dalley D and Boyd NF: The development of a method of

assessing the quality of life for cancer patients. Br J Cancer 1984 (20):849-859

64 Aaronson NK, Bullinger M and Ahmedzai S: A modular approach to quality of life assessment in cancer clinical trials. Recent Results in Cancer Res 1988 (111):231-249

65 Bergner M, Bobbitt Ra, Carter WB, and Gilson BS: The Sickness Impact Profile: Development and final revision of a health status measure. Med Care 1981 (19):787-805

66 Hunt SM, McKenna SP, McEwen J, Williams J and Papp E: The Nottingham Health Profile: Subjective health status and medical consultations. Soc Sci Med 1981 (15a):221-229

67 Anderson JP, Bush JW and Berry CC: Classifying function for health outcome and quality of life evaluation. Self versus individual models. Medical Care 1986 (24):454-469

68 Brook RH, Ware JE, Davies-Avery A et al.: Conceptualization and Measurement of Health for Adults in the Health Insurance Study: Vol VIII, Overview. Santa Monica, CA, The RAND Corporation, publication number R-1987/8-HEW 1979

69 Stewart AL, Hays RD and Ware JE: The MOS Short-form General Health Survey. Med Care 1988 (26):724-735

70 Feinstein AR: Clinimetric perspectives. J Chron Dis 1987 (40):635-640

71 Fallowfield L: Do psychological studies upset patients? In: Holland JC (ed) Syllabus of the Post-Graduate Course: Current Concepts in Psycho-Oncology and AIDS. Memorial Sloan-Kettering Cancer Center, New York 1987 p 335

V. Future Directions for Training and Research

Informed Consent and Cancer Clinical Research

Neil K. Aaronson [1] and Robert Zittoun [2]

1 Department of Psychosocial Research, The Netherlands Cancer Institute, Plesmanlaan 121, 1066 CX Amsterdam, The Netherlands

2 Service d'Hématologie, Hôtel Dieu, 1, Place du Parvis Notre Dame, 75181 Paris Cedex 04, France

Clinical trials represent an indispensable tool for testing, in a rigorous scientific manner, the efficacy of new cancer therapies. Without the cooperation of patients, such clinical trials would not be possible. The process of obtaining such cooperation - the informed consent process - has been the subject of increasing attention in recent years. Clinician-researchers, biomedical ethicists, lawmakers and social scientists have all entered the arena of debate regarding the need for, the effectiveness of, and the risks and benefits attached to informed consent procedures.

The moral and ethical foundation of informed consent can be traced to the promotion of two values: personal well-being and self-determination or autonomy [1,2]. The principal goal of the informed consent procedure is to provide a mechanism for patients to decide whether or not to participate in clinical research based on a full understanding of the factors relevant to that decision [3]. Meisel and Roth [4] describe informed consent as a process whereby "*information* is disclosed by a physician to a *competent* person, that person will *understand* the information and *voluntarily* make a *decision* to accept or refuse the recommended medical procedure."

Guidelines regarding informed consent for human experimentation have been internationally canonised in two documents: the 1948 Nuremberg Code and the 1964 Declaration of Helsinki. The Nuremberg Code, generated in response to the unprecedented abuses carried out by Nazi physicians during the Second World War, has as its first principle that the voluntary consent of the individual is "absolutely essential." The Code emphasises that such consent should be based on a knowledge and understanding of the proposed procedures, and of the potential risks involved in those procedures. The Helsinki Declaration, targetted toward *medical* research involving human subjects, outlines the specific topics that should be addressed during the informed consent procedure. These include: (a) the aims and methods of the research; (b) anticipated benefits and potential risks of the study; and (c) the right of the individual to refuse participation and to withdraw from the study at any time. Additionally, it is recommended that consent be obtained in writing.

The broad principles of informed consent embodied in the Nuremberg Code and the Declaration of Helsinki are the product of international consensus. Nevertheless, the *practice* of informed consent in medical research settings varies widely from country to country, from institution to institution within a given country, and even from physician to physician within a given institution.

The most formalised and standardised informed consent regulations can be found in the United States. Both federal and pharmaceutical industry regulations require that *written* informed consent be obtained from patients before they are entered into clinical trials. These U.S. requirements would appear to be motivated as much by legal as by ethical considerations. That is, the litigious nature of American society recommends the use of written informed consent procedures as a means of protecting both physicians and hospitals against potential law suits. This has resulted, in some cases, in the use of written materials that follow the letter, but not necessarily the spirit of informed consent.

In European countries, where malpractice claims are still relatively infrequent, one finds a greater variation in the form and content of informed consent procedures. Nevertheless, there is a clear trend toward adoption of the American model. Thus, in countries such as France and Holland, new legislation has been passed or is pending that would require written informed consent from patients asked to participate in clinical trials.

Despite the observable trend towards international standardisation of informed consent practices, the topic continues to engender a great deal of controversy. Its proponents insist that it is an essential mechanism for guarding individual rights in the medical context. Others are more skeptical, arguing that informed consent is a fiction; that patients do not understand, cannot understand, and do not want to be informed about experimental options, preferring instead to leave treatment decisions to their physician.

It is only relatively recently that the discussion surrounding the feasibility and effectiveness of informed consent procedures has been informed by empirical research. While it is beyond the scope of this paper to provide a comprehensive review of this body of literature, the most salient findings can be summarised as follows.

The large majority of patients appear to prefer open communication about their disease and to be fully informed about their treatment options, including how the choice of treatment is made [3-7]. Nevertheless, there remains a minority of patients who prefer only partial disclosure of information [8,9]. The question remains as to whether this latter group of patients should be considered ineligible for participation in clinical trials, or whether consent can also be accepted as legitimate even though patients prefer not to be fully informed.

It is unclear as to whether the informed consent process results in additional anxiety and distress among patients. While some studies indicate a short-term increase in distress as a result of full disclosure of information [10], others show no such effect [11], or even a lowering of distress levels [1]. Given the uncertainty surrounding this issue, one cannot take for granted the legitimacy of the concept of "therapeutic privilege" invoked frequently to justify the withholding of certain information in the interest of the patient's well-being.

Perhaps the most consistent finding to emerge from the research literature is that a significant percentage of patients entered into clinical trials are inadequately informed and/or cannot recall or understand important information with which they have been provided [4,5,7,13-16]. Younger patients, and those with higher educational levels tend to be better informed than older, less educated patients [7].

The provision of written information as a supplement to verbal explanations of treatment and trial procedures does not necessarily contribute to better patient knowledge and understanding [3,11,13,15,19]. Content analysis of informed consent forms has shown that they often have poor readability, sometimes with a difficulty level approaching that of professional medical journals [6,17,18]. The complexity of informed consent forms appears to result in cursory reading and inadequate recall [5].

A number of methods have been suggested for improving the effectiveness of informed consent procedures. These include:

a) providing simpler, more clearly written information to patients [6,18,20-23]
b) introducing a standard delay of several days between the patient's receipt of information and his/her decision whether or not to take part in a clinical trial [24];
c) employing videotape aids as an adjunct to verbal and written information [25];
d) providing educational programmes for physicians in communicating information to patients [1];
e) including other health care providers, and particularly the nursing staff, in the informed consent process [13,14,26];
f) having an "ombudsman" (i.e., someone familiar with the patient's situation, with expertise in oncology, and yet not personally involved in the proposed research) available to assure that patients have been adequately informed about a proposed protocol treatment, and to provide additional information where necessary [27,28].

While some of these proposed interventions have received empirical support, many have yet to be rigorously tested in applied clinical settings. In fact, there is a range of issues which deserves further attention in our effort to better understand and to enhance procedures for assuring optimal informed consent. As Meisel et al. [15] concluded in their review of empirical studies of the informed consent process: "What we find is that there is very little wheat and much chaff. Neither supporters nor detractors of the informed consent doctrine should find much comfort in the empirical literature; whether informed consent is feasible is still an open question."

Specifically, future research efforts should be directed toward determining:

a) factors related to variations in patients' desire for information regarding treatment and research options;
b) the patient, physician and clinical trial characteristics associated most closely with patients' level of knowledge and understanding of proposed protocol treatments;
c) the types of information that are better and less well understood by patients (i.e., disease, treatment or research-related information);
d) the role, if any, of "therapeutic privilege" in the informed consent process;
e) the feasibility and effectiveness of various (combinations of) interventions to enhance the informed consent process (preferably in the context of controlled studies).

The vast majority of research on informed consent undertaken has, to date, emanated from the United States. Given the increasing trend toward multi-centre, collaborative research, and the variability in ethical and legal standards and norms applied from country to country, it is essential that future studies in this area adopt a cross-cultural focus. As evidenced by the Nuremberg Code and the Declaration of Helsinki, it is possible to establish broad international consensus regarding the basic tenets applicable to informed consent in medical research. At the same time, however, we should not lose sight of the impact of culture on the ways in which such principles are interpreted and applied [29]. Finally, it should be emphasised that, regardless of the amount of empirical data that we generate, informed consent will remain an essentially moral and ethical problem [30]. At best, we can hope that such data will provide some guidance as to how we can best translate prevailing ethical standards and codes into viable practices and procedures.

REFERENCES

1 President's Commission for the Study of Ethical Problems in Medicine and Biomedical and Behavioral Research: Making Health Care Decisions: The Ethical and Legal Implications of Informed Consent in the Patient-Practitioner Relationship (Vol 1). US Government Printing Office, Washington DC 1982
2 Faden RR and Beauchamp TL: A History and Theory of Informed Consent. Oxford University Press, New York 1986
3 Cassileth BR, Zuphis RV, Sutton-Smith K et al: Information and participation preferences among cancer patients. Ann Intern Med 1980 (92):832-836
4 Meisel A and Rother LH: What we do and do not know about informed consent. JAMA 1981 (246):2473-2477
5 Cassileth BR, Zupkis RV, Sutton-Smith K and March V: Informed consent - Why are its goals imperfectly realized? N Engl J Med 1980 (302):896-900
6 White DR, Muss HB, Michielutte R et al: Informed consent: Patient information forms in chemotherapy trials. Am J Clin Oncol 1984 (7):183-190
7 Aaronson NK, van Dam FSAM, Visser-Pol GE et al: Informed consent and cancer clinical trials: A descriptive study. Report submitted on Project NKI 86-1 to the Dutch Cancer Society, Amsterdam, the Netherlands 1988
8 Christensen-Szalanski JJJ, Boyce WT, Harrel H and Gardner MM: Circumcision and informed consent: Is more information always better? Med Care 1987 (25):856-867
9 McIntosh J: Processes of communication, information seeking and control associated with cancer: A selective review of the literature. Soc Sci Med 1974 (8):167-175
10 Simes RJ, Tattersall MHN, Coates AS et al: Randomized comparison of procedures for obtaining informed consent in clinical trials of treatment for cancer. Br Med J 1986 (293):1065-1068
11 Dodd MJ: Measuring informational intervention for chemotherapy knowledge and self-care behavior. Res Nurs Hlth 1984 (7):43-50
12 Wallace LM: Psychological preparation as a method of reducing the stress of surgery. J Human Stress 1984 (10):62-77
13 Muss HB, White DR, Michielutte R et al: Written informed consent in patients with breast cancer. Cancer 1979 (43):1549-1566
14 Dodd MJ and Mood DW: Chemotherapy: Helping patients to know the drugs they are receiving and their possible side effects. Cancer Nurs 1981 (4):311-318
15 Penman DT, Holland JC, Bahna GF et al: Informed consent for investigational chemotherapy: Patients' and physicians' perceptions. J Clin Oncol 1984 (2):849-855
16 van Uden MMAT and van Dam FSAM: Informed consent bij klinisch kankeronderzoek; psychologische aspecten. Ned Tijdschr Geneesk 1986 (130):2078-2082
17 Morrow GR: How readable are subject consent forms? JAMA 1980 (244):56-58
18 Grundner TM: On the readability of surgical consent forms. N Engl J Med 1980 (302):900-902
19 Kennedy BJ and Lilehaugen A: Patient recall of informed consent. Med Pediatr Oncol 1979 (7):173-178
20 Schwalb E and Crosson K: Helping you help your patients: The patient education program of the National Cancer Institute. Oncol Nurs Forum 1988 (15):651-655
21 Ley P: Memory for medical information. Br J Soc Clin Psychol 1979 (18):245-255
22 Huchcroft S, Snodgrass T, Troyan S, Wares C: Testing the effectiveness of an information booklet for cancer patients. J Psychosoc Oncol 1984 (2):73-83
23 Tymchuk AJ, Ouslander JG and Rader N: Informing the elderly: A comparison of four methods. J Am Geriatr Soc 1986 (34):818-822
24 Morrow G, Gootnick J and Schmale A: A simple technique for increasing cancer patients' knowledge of informed consent to treatment. Cancer 1978 (42):793-799
25 Barbour GL and Blumenkrantz MJ: Videotape aids informed consent decision. JAMA 1978 (240):2741-2742
26 Rodenhuis S, van den Heuvel WJA, Annyas AA et al: Patient motivation and informed consent in a phase I study of an anticancer agent. Eur J Cancer Clin Oncol 1984 (20):457-462
27 Lincoln TL: Cancer decisions - What patients? The Rand Corporation, Santa Monica CA, 1978
28 van der Meer C: Informed consent: Een praktische benadering. Med Contact 1984 (43):1386-1288
29 Holland JC, Geary N, Marchini A and Tross S: An international survey of physicians attitudes and practice in regard to revealing the diagnosis of cancer. Cancer Invest 1987 (5):151-154
30 Zittoun R and Sancho-Garnier H: Ethical considerations for clinical trials in cancer patients. In: Rotmensz N (ed) Data Management and Clinical Trials. Elsevier Science Publishing, Amsterdam 1989 pp 37-48

Suicide and Euthanasia

Christina Bolund

Psychosocial Unit, Department of Oncology, Karolinska Hospital, S-104 01 Stockholm, Sweden

When healthy people confront the thought "If I get cancer", an immediate reaction is "I couldn't make it, I would take my life". Sometimes suicide is claimed to be the rational solution to cancer and terminal illness [1,2]. Yet very few cancer patients do commit suicide; in the few carefully performed epidemiological studies the rate of suicide in connection with cancer was found to be equal to or at the most double the rate among the healthy population [3-5]. These findings do not, however, preclude the possibility that the thought of suicide is a source of relief to many seriously ill patients threatened by powerlessness. The possibility of suicide means a way out, a means of regaining control.

When the factual and emotional circumstances around suicides committed by cancer patients are analysed, no simple pattern or "explanation" appears. One can see a mosaic of medical, psychiatric, social and psychological problems to which suicide was the patient's solution [6,7]. Some suicides are the reactions to an inner demand or distress, others are the response to the shortcomings of health care or the social network. Suicide should neither be viewed as the heroic choice of the strong, nor as the escape of the weak, but rather as a signal of loss of the meaning of life in the face of death or humiliation. The experience of trained psychotherapists is that a sense of meaning can be restored by human contact and open sharing of one's predicament [8].

Suicide is sometimes facilitated by relatives, friends, or health care staff [9]; in some countries it is permitted by law. Even the prescription of potentially lethal medication by physicians is not prohibited by law. In contrast, the active act of killing by injection of poisonous agents or the obstruction of airways is considered murder, irrespective of the state of health or the wish of the victim. In some European countries, there is a tendency to withhold punishment for acts of killing when the victim has been severely ill and has expressed a wish for mercy killing. In West Germany this tendency does not only concern the killing of terminally ill persons. A doctor was relieved of punishment in state court proceedings for killing a patient with a disfiguring tumour of the face by cyanide.

In several countries associations (often called Exit) were set up to plead for legislation permitting active euthanasia. In the Netherlands a Government committee in the early 1980s passed a law in favour of euthanasia which, however, was stopped in order to await the election of the new parliament. The proposed law was not passed by the new Government.

The provisional documents show a gradual shift in the proposed indications for euthanasia. Originally, very rigid requirements were considered the prerequisite for euthanasia: terminal illness (with only days of expected life), inability to commit suicide, the pronounced wish to die by active euthanasia, and scrutiny by a committee of two physicians and a priest. Several other proposed indications were presented, such as situations of longstanding debilitating disease with no requirement of conscious expression of the wish to be killed. This clearly illustrates the kind of difficulty that one encounters when trying to set principles in a human area too subtle to allow legislation. Many of those opposing the demand of legislation fear that any legislation will open the door to cynical, super-rational reasoning when dealing with human values and goals in terminal care. As yet it is only the Nazi government that has permitted euthanasia by law, a law that was in operation for less than one year. During that time it allowed the killing of thousands of severely and chronically ill, as well as psychiatric and mentally retarded patients.

An active spokesman for euthanasia in the Netherlands, the anaesthesiologist Pieter Admiraal, has claimed that yearly about 4,000 people, mostly cancer patients, die through euthanasia in his country, amounting to about 3% of all deaths. If this information is correct there is already without legislation a death industry within the health care system in Holland. No legal action has been taken against Dr. Admiraal or other physicians declaring that they perform euthanasia. On the other hand, four nurses admitting the killing of a senile patient were sentenced to prison. We hereby approach another key question for the advocates of euthanasia - which profession would be selected by society to take on the professional duty of killing? Mostly, it seems tacitly understood that it should be the responsibility of physicians. It has been suggested to give postgraduate courses providing physicians with knowledge on lethal doses and special ethical and psychological expertise not usually in their possession. Why are doctors proposed and not priests, nurses, psychologists, or judges - all professionals respected for their judgment in human matters?

It could very well be argued that for this kind of very sensitive decisions society might institute a profession of utmost specialisation in human psychology and ethics which, under the supervision of Parliament, would take on the duty to judge in life and death matters. Maybe it is significant that it is fiction writers who have taken the closest look at the consequences of legislation on euthanasia for humanism and human politics in the future [10]. An analysis of the psychological and ethical aspects of euthanasia is of need within the health care system [11].

REFERENCES

1 Choron J: Suicide. An Incisive Look at Self-Destruction. Charles Scribner's Sons, New York 1972

2 Kastenbaum P: Suicide as the preferred way of death. In: Schneidman JE (ed) Suicidology: Contemporary Developments. Grune & Stratton, New York 1976

3 Fox BH et al: Suicide rates among cancer patients in Connecticut. J Chron Dis 1982 (35):85-100

4 Louhivuori KA et al: Risk of suicide among cancer patients. Am J Epid 1979 (109):59-65

5 Allebeck P et al: Incidence of suicide among cancer patients in Sweden. Am J Epid 1989 (in press)

6 Bolund C: Suicide and Cancer. I. Demographical and suicidological description of cuicides among cancer patients in Sweden. J Psychosoc Oncol 1985 (3):17-30

7 Bolund C: Suicide and cancer. II. Medical and care factors in suicides by cancer patients in Sweden. J Psychosoc Oncol 1983 (3):31-52

8 Feigenberg L: Terminal Care. On Friendship Contracts with Dying Cancer Patients. Brunner/Mazel, New York 1980

9 Rollin B: Last Wish. Simon & Shuster, New York 1985

10 Huxley A: Brave New World. London 1932

11 Razavi D et al: Les euthanasies: Intrications des dimensions bioéthiques et psychologiques. Ann Med Psychol (Paris) 1987 (145):833-848

Unorthodox Cancer Treatments

Neil K. Aaronson[1] and Jimmie C. Holland [2]

1 Department of Psychosocial Research, The Netherlands Cancer Institute, Plesmanlaan 121, 1066 CX Amsterdam, The Netherlands
2 Psychiatry Service, Memorial Sloan-Kettering Cancer Center, 1275 York Avenue, New York, NY 10021, USA

The use of unorthodox (also termed "unconventional", "alternative" or "unproven") treatments among cancer patients is the subject of widespread and often heated debate. Proponents of unorthodox treatments argue that they offer patients the opportunity to participate actively in their fight against cancer, that they facilitate improved resistance, both physically and psychologically, to disease symptoms and conventional treatment side effects, and that they contribute to the control or even to the cure of the disease. Those opposed to unorthodox therapies are concerned that they give patients false hope and that they may, implicitly or explictly, encourage non-adherence to or outright rejection of conventional oncological treatments.

The proliferation of modern unorthodox cancer therapies should not be viewed as an isolated, aberrant phenomenon. Alternative approaches to normative medical practice date back to the early 19th century. As Cassileth and Brown [1] point out, unproven medical remedies thrive in the face of incurable disease. In the 19th century, it was tuberculosis which stimulated the market for unorthodox treatments. When an effective treatment for that disease was discovered, the market for unproven remedies evaporated. Today, cancer provides the breeding ground for the alternative medicine circuit. While optimistic official figures suggest that the "war on cancer" is being won, other evidence indicates that, for the major forms of cancer (lung, breast, gastrointestinal), the survival rates have not improved significantly during the past quarter century [2]. This fact, combined with the more anecdotal forms of information readily available to cancer patients and their families (e.g., reports in the press of the cancer-related death of celebrities and other public figures), creates a climate of uncertainty conducive to experimentation with alternative forms of treatment.

Despite the extensive public debate surrounding unorthodox cancer treatments, it is only recently that serious efforts have been undertaken to document the prevalence with which such therapies are used and to investigate the motives underlying their use. With regard to the prevalence of use, estimates range between less than 10% [3] to more than 50% of patients [4]. This wide range in prevalence figures may reflect true differences related to the cultural composition of the study samples (i.e., the use of alternative treatments does not appear to be consistent across countries). Various conceptual and methodological factors can also influence prevalence estimates. For example, studies differ in the definitional boundaries that they employ to distinguish between conventional and non-conventional forms of treatment, as well as in the sources that they draw upon to accrue their study samples (e.g., the records of conventional cancer centres versus those of alternative practitioners).

Many of the unorthodox therapies used by cancer patients are based on the same fundamental premise - that cancer is caused by a disturbance of the natural metabolic balance, and that cure is possible through a restoration of that balance. Given this starting point, however, a wide variety of alternative therapies are available which differ in terms of diagnostic and treatment methods. In the United States, these include metabolic therapy (a combination of special diet, vitamins and minerals), diet treatments, megavitamins, mental imagery, spiritual or faith-healing, and "immune" therapy [5]. In Germany, beet juice and mistletoe (Iscador) are commonly used [6]. In Holland, the large majority of patients who pursue unorthodox treatment follow the "Moerman diet" [7]. In Finland, extract of birch root is frequently used [8].

Research into the use of unorthodox cancer therapies has dispelled a number of misconceptions surrounding the characteristics of the user group, and the motives associated with their use. Contrary to popular belief, the modal user of unorthodox therapies is not a terminally ill, poorly educated patient who is "grasping at straws" in the search for effective treatment. Rather, patients are often well-educated and in either an early disease stage or in remission [4].

The available evidence suggests that the decision to use an unorthodox therapy is motivated by both a dissatisfaction with conventional cancer treatment, and an attraction to a number of elements found commonly in alternative treatment approaches [5,7]. In particular, alternative therapeutic approaches often offer patients a more active role in their treatment and a closer doctor-patient relationship than is typically the case within the conventional health care system. Further, while the clinical efficacy of alternative cancer therapies is unproven, only infrequently do they carry with them serious risks of physical harm (see ref. 9 for exceptions). Their generally benign nature is in sharp contrast to the toxicities associated frequently with aggressive conventional treatment.

Awareness of the positive characteristics frequently attributed to unorthodox therapies provides a number of important leads as to how conventional care of cancer patients might be improved. First, greater attention could be devoted to conveying one's concern with the patient's overall well-being (i.e., quality of life), rather than focusing narrowly on the biology of the disease. Second, patients could be offered a more active role in their own health care. For example, Cassileth [1] suggests that providing patients with reasonable dietary guidelines might diffuse the attractiveness of alternative therapies that offer such self-care elements. Finally, there should be a greater willingness to discuss openly with patients the pros and cons of adopting unorthodox cancer therapies. A rigid, anti-alternative treatment stance will only encourage patients to seek advice and council outside of the conventional health care system.

In terms of future research efforts, there are at least two areas that deserve further attention. First, it would be extremely useful to undertake a collaborative, international survey of the attitudes and practices of cancer patients, conventional care-givers, and unorthodox practitioners with regard to alternative cancer treatments. By employing a standard conceptual and methodological framework in such a cross-cultural undertaking, it would be possible to reconcile a number of the conflicting results that have emerged from studies undertaken to date. Additionally, the use of general theoretical models of health and illness behaviour and of coping with chronic disease in such research could shed more light on the complex of factors related to the use of unorthodox cancer therapies.

Second, it would be useful to carry out controlled clinical trials of selective unorthodox therapies. Clearly, such an undertaking is beset with ethical, political and practical problems. On the one hand, there is a reluctance on the part of the practitioners of unorthodox treatments to submit their techniques to classical experimental investigation. On the other hand, legitimate voices of protest are raised within the conventional medical establishment regarding the ethics of randomising patients to receive an unorthodox therapy.

Nevertheless, in selective situations (e.g., adjuvant treatment settings), these obstacles can be successfully overcome. For example, the EORTC Melanoma Cooperative Group is currently conducting a phase III clinical trial to evaluate the efficacy of low-dose, long-term treatment with alpha or gamma-interferon as an adjuvant (i.e., post-surgical) treatment for patients with stage I or stage IIb malignant melanoma with unfavourable prognosis [10]. In this trial, an optional treatment arm to which patients can be randomised involves the administration of Iscador. To our knowledge, this is the first controlled study to be conducted by a recognised clinical trials group in which an unorthodox therapy is included as one of the treatment arms. In the long run, it is through such efforts that the rhetoric surrounding the topic of unorthodox therapies can be replaced by reasoned argument.

REFERENCES

1 Cassileth BR and Brown: Unorthodox cancer medicine. Cancer 1988 (38):176-187

2 Bailar JC and Smith EM: Progress against cancer? N Engl J Med 1986 (314):1226-1232

3 Eidenger RW and Shapiro DV: Cancer patients insight into their treatment prognosis and unconventional therapies. Cancer 1984 (53):2736-2740

4 Cassileth BR, Lusk EJ, Strouse TB and Bodenheimer BA: Contemporary unorthodox treatments in cancer medicine. Ann Internal Med 1984 (101):105-112

5 Cassileth BR: Unorthodox Cancer Medicine. Cancer Invest 1986 (4):591-598

6 Obrist R, von Meiss M and Obrecht JP: Verwendung paramedizinisher behandlungsmethoden durch tumorpatienten. Deutsche Medizinische Wochenschrift 1986 (111):283-287

7 Reurink I, van der Zouwe N, van Dam FSAM, Aaronson NK, Rumke P and Hanewald GJPF: Concurrent use of unorthodox and conventional cancer therapies. Satellite Symposia Proc, ECCO-4 1987:24.

8 Arkko PJ, Arkko BT, Kari-Koskinen L and Taskinen PJ: A survey of unproven cancer remedies and their use in an outpatient clinic for cancer therapy in Finland. Soc Sci Med 1980 (14a):511-514

9 Markman M: Medical complications of "alternative" cancer therapy. N Engl J Med 1985 (312):1640-1641

10 Kleeberg UR: EORTC protocol 18871: Adjuvant trial in malignant melanoma comparing interferon r alpha-2 to r gamma to a control group after surgical removal of either high risk primary or curative resection of lymph node metastasis. EORTC Data Center, Brussel 1988

Psychoneuroimmunological Studies

Marzio Sabbioni [1] and Christoph Hürny [2]

1 University Psychiatry Department, Murtenstrasse 21, 3010 Bern, Switzerland
2 Medical Department C.L. Lory, Inselspital Bern, Freiburgstrasse, 3010 Bern, Switzerland

Current Knowledge

The interactions between the central nervous system and the immune system have received increasing attention in the last years [1-3]. It has been shown that lymph nodes, thymus and spleen are innervated with sympathetic nerves. This innervation regulates not only the blood flow but also the immune function of these organs [4-8]. Induction of an immune response has been shown to correlate with increased firing rates of hypothalamic neurons, while lesion or stimulation of various central nervous system areas, particularly within the hypothalamus, result in altered immune response: suppression of an anaphylactic reaction, reduced stimulation of T-cell lymphocytes with mitogens, reduced or abolished Natural Killer cell activity [9-13]. These results support the assumption of a direct link between the nervous system and the immune system.
The interactions between the endocrine system and the immune system have also been investigated [3,24]: lymphocytes and granulocytes bear receptors for hormones, neurotransmitters and neuropeptides. The immunosuppressive effect of glucocorticosteroids in pharmacological doses is well known. Adrenalin in physiological doses increases the Natural Killer cell activity [25] or the number and activity of circulating suppressor T-cells.
The interaction of psychosocial factors with the immune system has been investigated by several research groups in experimental animals and in humans. Rather than a comprehensive overview, some examples will be presented here.
Classical conditioning can modify immune responses [14-18]. This has been shown repeatedly in experimental animals. The delayed hypersensitivity reaction to tuberculin in humans was reduced following a paradigm similar to behavioural conditioning [19].
The interaction of presumably "psychic" stress with the immune system in experimental animals has been shown in several studies [20]. The stressors were overcrowding, restraint, shocks or noise.The difficulty in this research is how to define a "psychic" stressor for animals (are electroshocks a psychic stressor?). Besides these problems, one of the most interesting results for our discussion is that animals who had control over the stressor had less immunosuppression [21], or died later because of slower tumour growth [22], or could defend themselves better against tumour induction [23].
The influence of stress and emotions like anxiety or depression on immune function has also been investigated in humans [2,24,25]. Some of the first investigations were done in spaceflight research [29] and in a laboratory with sleep deprivation and noise as stressors [30].
The results of epidemiologic studies showing higher mortality and morbidity in bereaved spouses led to the investigation of the immune system in bereavement [31-33]. The response of lymphocytes to phytohaemagglutinin (PHA) and to concanavalin A (con A) was significantly depressed in bereaved spouses compared to a non-bereaved control group [31]. Bereaved women had significantly lower Natural Killer cell activity than women whose

husbands were healthy. The symptoms of depression are related to a reduction in Natural Killer cell activity during bereavement [32]. In another study, the effect of depressed mood on immune status (lymphocyte reactivity measured by mixed lymphocyte culture and lymphocyte response to PHA) was considerably greater in subjects that had experienced a recent death or serious family illness [28].

The studies linking stressful life changes to disease onset opened another field for psychoneuroimmunological studies. The results are contradictory. The antibody response to influenza vaccination showed no relation to life change stress in some studies [34,35]. In another study, there was a relation between the antibody rise and the amount of life change stress and the coping abilities [25]. In this study and in others, poor copers under stress showed a reduced Natural Killer cell activity. In reviewing these studies, Locke [25] raises the important question of time in these processes: "(The) differences in the relationship of time of immune function and life stress time frame raise interesting speculations about possible differential susceptibility of the humoral and cellular components of the immune system to the effects of acute or chronic stress".

Significant changes in immune function were shown when college examinations were investigated as a stressor [36-44]: decrease in Natural Killer cell activity [36], decreased proliferative response of lymphocytes [37], smaller percentage of helper T-lymphocytes without significant change in the ratio of suppressor T-lymphocytes [38], increase in antibody titers to Epstein-Barr virus [39], depressed interferon production by Con A-stimulated leukocytes [40].

Similar studies have been performed in psychiatric patients [26,45-47], showing a reduced lymphocyte responsiveness to mitogen (Con A and PHA) in depressive disorders or in mania. In another study on psychiatric patients, severe loneliness was associated with significantly lower Natural Killer cell activity, as well as poor T-lymphocyte response to PHA [48].

The role of interpersonal relationships in immune function has been investigated in patients with marital disruption and caregivers of relatives with Alzheimer's disease. Immune changes (number and function of Natural Killer cells, percentage of T-helper-lymphocytes) were related to loneliness, attachment and depression [49-51]. Unemployed women showed a decrease of the reactivity of lymphocytes to purified protein derivative (PPD) of tuberculin and to PHA [52].

The relationship between personality traits and immunity has also been investigated. Higher need for succorance/nurturance was associated with a drop in the helper/inducer T-lymphocyte counts, whereas more achievement- and order-oriented subjects showed higher suppressor/cytotoxic T-lymphocyte counts under the stress of a five-day self-awareness course [53].

To sum up, there is now much evidence for relationships between psychosocial factors and immunological functions. *In vitro* measures of cellular immune function such as Natural Killer cell activity or lymphoblast transformation are suppressed in an individual who is distressed, lonely or depressed or who is a poor coper when experiencing high life change stress. There also appear to be links between humoral immunity and psychosocial factors, but the results are more controversial. Subjects having a chronic viral infection with Epstein-Barr virus, Cytomegalovirus or Herpes simplex virus have higher specific antibodies when under stress. This could be a compensatory mechanism of the humoral immune function because of the suppressed cellular immune function under stress.

The Interest of Psychooncology in Psychoneuroimmunology

The immune system probably plays an important role in the development of cancer and in its treatment. The immunosurveillance hypothesis postulates a failure of the immune system to control development and spread of malignant cells. The Natural Killer cells are thought to play an important role together with other effector cells: cytotoxic T-cell, antibody-dependent cell cytotoxicity, cytotoxic effects of monocytes by Tumour Necrosis Factor. There is an interaction with regulator cells such as monocytes, T4-lymphocytes by cell-to-cell contact or short distance messengers like in-

terleukines. T8-lymphocytes and the anti-idiotypic immune response act as counterregulation.
Immunological problems also play an important role in the treatment of cancer. Chemotherapy, radiotherapy and probably cancer itself have cytotoxic and immunosuppressive side effects limiting the use of these agents or causing serious complications, such as infections.
As discussed in a previous chapter of this monograph, the influence of psychosocial factors in cancer risk and survival has been extensively studied. But there are only few studies investigating specifically the link between psychosocial factors, immune status and cancer. In a very interesting study of patients with early breast cancer, tumour burden was associated with Natural Killer cell activity and a significant proportion of Natural Killer cell activity level variance could be predicted by patients' "adjustment, lack of social support and fatigue/depression symptoms" [54, 55].
A better knowledge of the relationship between psychosocial factors and immune system could enable us to recognise individuals at risk for cancer or for side effects of cancer treatment, and to plan effective interventions. Unfortunately, we are still far away from these possibilities.

Methodological Problems in Psychoneuroimmunological Studies

Different Views on the Relationship between Psychological and Biological Processes

There are only few authors who, at the beginning of a study, explicitly mention their understanding of the relationship between psychological and biological processes. Because this relationship could not be explained scientifically up to now, we have to use and explain our bias concerning this matter. The different ways of thinking cannot be extensively discussed here, but they may have a substantial influence on the hypothesis and the research methods. Psychological and biological processes may be conceived, for instance, as complementary, identical or as a dialectic entity. Some researchers may use cybernetic concepts in order to understand this relationship. These are only some examples to illustrate the current range of the ideas about this problem.

Assessing Multiple Aspects of Life Processes

In psychoimmunological research, emotional, behavioural and immunological processes are assessed simultaneously by different methods. Implicitly there is the assumption that it is possible to describe the psychological and immunological phenomena within a model of linear correlations.
There is a better correlation of psychosocial and immunological data when measurements are performed within the individual over time than in an interindividual comparison. Many questions are raised by this fact: Is the model of linear correlations adequate to describe these phenomena? What is the importance of time frame of psychological and physiological processes? Are the investigated processes specific for the individual or for the stimulus? What is the influence of the psychosocial and immunological base-line values?
This applies also to the relationships between psychosocial factors, immune system and cancer. The links may be still more complicated because three elements have to be studied at the same time.
In psychoimmunological research a choice has to be made between a great number of parameters that could be measured or assessed. In order to have the possibility to compare the results, there is a need to define specific relevant experimental settings, specific relevant phenomena to investigate and specific relevant questions to be answered.

The Measurement of Psychosocial and Immunological Factors

Is it ethical to use the chosen investigational methods in human research? Are they close to everyday life? Do they only have a minimal influence on the studied process? Are they acceptable for patients/subjects? Is it possible to use them on a large scale? Are they suitable for multivariate analysis? These questions have to be raised while designing a new study.

A wide range of distinct methods have been used so far. Therefore it is difficult to compare the studies and to draw generally accepted conclusions. The results stand by themselves and cannot be integrated into a concept.

Several serious attempts have been made to measure "stress" and emotions such as "anxiety", but a good standard does not exist. There are also difficulties to assess depressed mood, because the known depression scales were constructed to assess depression as a psychiatric syndrome. To make the different studies more comparable it would be useful to use multiple methods to measure one psychosocial factor.

In psychoimmunological studies only a limited number of measurements of the immunological functions is possible. The timing of the different measurements has to be defined very clearly. The fact that only punctual measurements are possible raises the question as to how to assess a relationship between immunological functions and psychosocial factors over time. Immunological functions have considerable interindividual variance and may react to multiple influences such as a sun bath, physical activity, nutrition, sleep and others. Assessment of Natural Killer cell activity or stimulation with Con A or PHA are widely used as indicators of the immune status. These laboratory examinations are complicated. The values depend upon many laboratory factors. Furthermore, they are *in vitro* measures and there remain questions as tohow well they reflect the immune status *in vivo*. It is still controversial whether the statistical differences found in different studies of these immune functions are of any biological (clinical) relevance. This has to be proved by prospective clinical studies. *In vivo* measures of immune functions that are simple and applicable on a large scale have to be found. Perhaps the assessment of lymphokines could be helpful for this purpose.

What Needs to be Done?

A great effort is necessary to clarify different methodological problems in psychoimmunological research. Valid and reliable methods have to be developed to measure emotions, behaviour and immunological functions; methods that can be used on a large scale, are close to everyday life, have little influence on the measured functions and are suitable for multivariate analysis. The problem of time frame of emotions, behaviour, immunological functions and illness has to be studied more closely. The question whether it is correct to assume that the relationship between psychosocial and immunological functions and cancer can be described with a model of linear correlations should be approached on a more basic level of understanding life processes. However, at the current state of research, it is the only generally accepted model. The clinical relevance of the results has to be investigated, not only postulated on the basis of theoretical assumptions.

REFERENCES

1 Ader R (ed): Psychoneuroimmunology. Academic Press, New York 1981

2 Schulz K-H and Rädler A: Tumorimmunologie und Psychoimmunologie als Grundlagen für die Psychoonkologie. Psychother med Psychol 1986 (36):114-129

3 Fox BH and Newberry BH (eds): Impact of Psychoendocrine Systems in Cancer and Immunity. CJHogrefe, Lewinston 1984

4 Felten DL, Felten SY, Bellinger DL, Carlson SL, Ackerman KD, Madden KS, Olschowki and Livnat S: Noradrenergic sympathetic neural interactions with the immune system: Structure and function. Immunol Rev 1987 (100):225-260

5 Giron LT, Crutcher KA and Davis JN: Lymph nodes - a possible site for sympathetic neuronal regulation of immune responses. Ann Neurol 1980 (8):520-525

6 Williams JM and Felten DL: Sympathetic innervation of murine thymus and spleen. A comparative histofluorescence study. Anatom Rec 1981 (199):531-542

7 Williams JM, Peterson RG, Shea PA, Schmedtje JF, Bauer DC and Felten DL: Sympathetic innervation of murine thymus and spleen. Evidence for a functional link between the nervous and immune systems. Brain Res Bull 1981 (6):83-84

8 Bulloch K and Moore RY: Innervation of the thymus gland by brain stem and spinal cord in mouse and rat. Am J Anat 1981 (162):157-166

9 Stein M, Keller S and Schleifer S: The hypothalamus and the immune response. In: Weiner H, Hofer MA, Stunkard AJ (eds) Brain, Behavior and Bodily Disease. Raven Press, New York 1981

10 Renoux G, Biziere K, Bardos P, Degenne D and Renoux M: NK activity in mice is controlled by the brain neocortex. In: Herberman RB (ed) NK Cells and Other Natural Effector Cells. Academic Press, New York 1982

11 Renoux G, Biziere K, Renoux M and Guillaumin JM: The production of T-cell-inducing factors in mice is controlled by the brain neocortex. Scand J Immunol 1983 (17):45-50

12 Renoux G, Biziere K, Guillaumin JM and Degenne D: A balanced brain asymmetry modulates T-cell-mediated events. J Neuroimmunol 1983 (5):227-238

13 Forni G., Bindoni M , Santoni A, Belluardo N, Marchese AE and Giovarelli M: Radiofrequency destruction of the tuberoinfundibular region of hypothalamus permanently abrogates NK Cell activity in mice. Nature 1983 (306):181-184

14 Bovbjerg D and Ader R: The central nervous system and learning: Feedforward regulation of immune responses. In: Berczi I (ed) Pituitary Function and Immunity. CRC Press, Boca Raton FL 1986 pp 251-259

15 Ader R and Cohen N: Behaviourally conditioned immunosuppression. Psychosom Med 1975 (37):333-340

16 Bovbjerg D, Ader R and Cohen N: Acquisition and extinction of a graft-vs-host response in the rat. J Immunol 1984 (132):111-113

17 Bovbjerg D, Cohen N and Ader R: The central nervous system and learning: A strategy for immune regulation. Immunol Today 1982 (3):287-291

18 Rogers MP, Reich P, Storm TB and Carpenter CB: Behaviourally conditioned immunosuppression: Replication of a recent study. Psychosom Med 1976 (38):447-451

19 Smith GR and McDaniel S: Psychological mediated effect on the delayed hypersensitivity reaction to Tuberculin in humans. Psychosom Med 1983 (45):65-70

20 Borysenko M and Borysenko J: Stress behavior and immunity: Animal models and mediating mechanisms. Gen Hosp Psych 1982 (4):59-67

21 Laudenslager ML, Ryan SM, Drugan RC, Hyson RL and Maier SF: Coping and immunosuppression: Inescapable but not escapable shock suppresses lymphocyte proliferation. Science 1983 (221):568-570

22 Sklar LS and Anisman H: Stress and coping factors influence tumor growth. Science 1979 (205):513-515

23 Visintainer MA, Volpicelli JR and Seligman MEP: Tumor rejection in rats after inescapable or escapable shock. Science 1982 (216):437-439

24 Calabrese JR, Kling MA and Gold PW: Alterations in immunocompetence during stress, bereavement and depression: Focus on neuroendocrine regulation. Am J Psychiatry 1987 (144):1123-1134

25 Locke SE: Stress, adaptation and immunity: Studies in humans. Gen Hosp Psych 1982 (4):49-58

26 Stein M, Keller SE and Schleifer SJ: Stress and immunomodulation: The role of depression and neuroendocrine function. J Immunol 1985 (135):827s-833s

27 Locke SE, Kraus L, Leserman J, Hurst MW, Heisel JS and Williams RM: Life change stress, psychiatric symptoms, and Natural Killer cell activity. Psychosom Med 1984 (46):441-453

28 Linn W, Linn BS and, Jensen J: Stressful events, dysphoric mood and immune responsiveness. Psychol Rep 1984 (54):219-222

29 Fischer CL, Daniels JC, Levin WC, Kimzey SL, Cobb EK and Ritzmann SE: Effects of the space flight environment on man's immune system: II. Lymphocyte counts and reactivity. Aerospace Med 1972 (43):1122-1125

30 Palmblad J, Petrini B, Wassermann J and Ackerstedt T: Lymphocyte and granulocyte reactions during sleep deprivation. Psychosom Med 1979 (41):273-278

31 Bartrop RW, Luckhurst E, Lazarus L, Kiloh LG and Penny R: Depressed lymphocyte function after bereavement. Lancet 1977 (1):834-836

32 Irwin M, Daniels M, Smith TL, Bloom E and Weiner H: Impaired Natural Killer cell activity during bereavement. Brain Behav Immunol 1987 (1): 98-104

33 Schleifer SJ, Keller SE, Camerino M, Thornton JC and Stein M: Suppression of lymphocyte stimulation following bereavement. JAMA 1983 (250):374-377

34 Locke SE and Heisel JS: The influence of stress and emotions on human immunity. (Abstract) Biofeed Self Regul 1977 (2):320

35 Greene WA, Betts RF, Ochitill HN, Iker HP and Douglas RG: Psychosocial factors and immunity:

Preliminary report. (Abstract) Psychosom Med 1978 (40):87
36 Kiecolt-Glaser JK, Garner W, Speicher S, Penn GM, Holliday J and Glaser R: Psychosocial modifiers of immunocompetence in medical students. Psychosom Med 1984 (46):7-14
37 Halvorsen R and Vassend O: Effects of examination stress on some cellular immunity functions. J Psychosom Res 1987 (31):693-701
38 Kiecolt-Glaser JK, Glaser R, Strain EC, Stout JC, Tarr KL, Holliday JE and Speicher CE: Modulation of cellular immunity in medical students. J Behav Med 1986 (9):5-21
39 Glaser R, Rice J, Sheridan J, Fertel R, Stout J, Speicher C, Pinsky D, Kotur M, Post A, Beck M and Kiecolt-Glaser J: Stress-related immune suppression: Health implications. Brain Behav Immunol 1987 (1):7-20
40 Glaser R, Rice J, Speicher CE, Stout JC and Kiecolt-Glaser JK: Stress depresses interferon production by leukocytes concomitant with a decrease in Natural Killer cell activity. Behav Neuroscience 1986 (100):675-678
41 Vassend O and Halvorsen R: Personality, examination stress and serum concentration of immunoglobulins. Scand J Psychol 1987 (28):233-241
42 Dorian B, Garfinkel P, Brown G, Shore A, Gladman D and Keystone E: Aberrations in lymphocyte subpopulations and function during psychological stress. Clin Exp Immunol 1982 (50):132-138
43 Glaser R, Kiecolt-Glaser JK, Stout JC, Tarr KL, Speicher CE and Holliday JE: Stress-related impairments in cellular immunity. Psychiat Res 1985 (16):233-239
44 Glaser R, Kiecolt-Glaser JK, Speicher CE and Holliday JE: Stress, loneliness and changes in Herpes virus latency. J Behav Med 1985 (8):249-260
45 Schleifer SJ, Keller SE, Meyerson AT, Raskin MJ, Davis KL and Stein M: Lymphocyte function in major depressive disorder. Arch Gen Psychiatry 1984 (41):484-486
46 Schleifer SJ, Keller SE, Siris SG, Davis KL and Stein M: Depression and immunity. Lymphocyte function in ambulatory depressed, hospitalized schizophrenic and herniorraphy patients. Arch Gen Psychiat 1985 (42):129-133
47 Kronfol Z and House JD: Immune function in mania. Biol Psychiat 1988 (24):341-343
48 Kiecolt-Glaser JK, Ricker D, George J, Messick G, Speicher CE, Garner W and Glaser R: Urinary cortisol levels, cellular immunocompetency, and loneliness in psychiatric inpatients. Psychosom Med 1984 (46):15-23
49 Kennedy S, Kiecolt-Glaser JK and Glaser R: Immunological consequences of acute and chronic stressors: Mediating role of interpersonal relationships. Br J Med Psychol 1988 (61):77-85
50 Kiecolt-Glaser JK, Fisher LD, Ogrocki P, Stout JC, Speicher CE and Glaser R: Marital quality, marital disruption, and immune function. Psychosom Med 1987 (49):13-34
51 Kiecolt-Glaser JK, Glaser R, Shuttleworth EC, Dyer CS, Ogrocki P and Speicher CE: Chronic stress and immunity in family caregivers of Alzheimer's disease victims. Psychosom Med 1987 (49):523-535
52 Arnetz BB, Wasserman J, Petrini B, Brenner SO, Levi L, Eneroth P, Salovaara H, Hjelm R, Salovaara L, Theorell T and Petterson IL: Immune function in unemployed women. Psychosom Med 1987 (49):3-12
53 Kropiunigg U, Hamilton G, Roth E and Simmel A: Selektive Wirkung von Persönlichkeitsmerkmalen und psychosozialem Stress auf die T-Lymphocyten-Subpopulationen. Psychother med Psychol 1989 (39):18-25
54 Levy S, Herberman R, Lippman M and d'Angelo T: Correlation of stress factors with sustained depression of Natural Killer cell activity and predicted prognosis in patients with breast cancer. J Clin Oncol 1987 (5):348-353
55 Levy SM, Herberman RB, Maluish AM, Schlien B and Lippman M: Prognostic risk assessment in primary breast cancer by behavioral and immunological parameters. Health Psychol 1985 (4):99-113

Psychological Sequelae in Cancer Survivors

Jimmie C. Holland

Psychiatry Service, Memorial Sloan-Kettering Cancer Center, 1275 York Avenue, New York, NY 10021, USA

Psychological problems of cancer survivors have added a new dimension to psychooncology research, as more patients, particularly young ones, survive and return to a normal life. However, they are usually concerned about psychosocial problems which impact on quality of life. These are: fears associated with termination of treatment; fears of recurrence or second malignancy; adaptation to "unanticipated" late effects (infertility, CNS dysfunction, organ failure); chronic stress on patient and family; development of "survivor" syndrome (guilt); and adaptation to negative social responses (job, coworkers and friends). The latter impinges heavily on the ability to change jobs, attain promotions and, in the United States, obtain health insurance. For a detailed review of the issues briefly mentioned here, see Tross and Holland [1].

Our observations of patients finishing radiotherapy treatments revealed an unexpected and significant increase in psychological distress at the *end* of treatment. The separation from checkups by the doctor and the perceived stopping of the protective effects of the treatment contribute to increased anxiety. The even more difficult question of *when* maintenance therapy, particularly in leukaemia, should end, is another source of fear. Patients continue years later to experience anxiety when minor symptoms (which earlier would have been ignored) develop.

Adaptation to the possibility of delayed side effects of treatment constitutes part of the medically-related concerns which directly affect quality of life. Fear of the risk of a second malignancy caused by treatment, neurotoxicity, damage to renal and cardiovascular systems, and infertility caused by chemotherapeutic agents and/or radiation alter normal function and thus cause emotional distress. Ovarian failure related to chemotherapy regimens account for diminished libido and sexual dysfunction in a high percentage of young women following the MOPP regimen for Hodgkin's disease and adjuvant chemotherapy in breast cancer. Frequently, women have not been prepared for this treatment-related early menopause, and an explanation of hormonal replacement therapy can be helpful.

Men also experience high frequency of sterility with the MOPP regimen in Hodgkin's disease. Men who receive unshielded pelvic radiation become aspermic after 3-4 treatments and remain sterile. While retroperitoneal node dissection for testicular neoplasms causes no loss in sexual performance, ejaculation is impaired and sterility may result due to interruption of the sympathetic chain. Sperm banking should be an integral part of management to make the adjustment to later infertility easier.

The psychosocial issue which all face is a diminished sense of self-confidence and of security about the future. This impinges on the ability to function well in the family and at work. Oncologists can help during treatment to alleviate these problems by bearing in mind several principles:

1. Honesty about the diagnosis; clear communication between the physician, patient and family about diagnosis, treatment and expectations.
2. Honesty about possible long-term adverse side effects. Unanticipated side effects, especially infertility, are easier to accept if planned for and expected.
3. Support of patients as active treatment terminates and heightened anxiety may occur.

4. Continuity of the treating physician and staff. The complexity of cancer treatments requires that many consultants and specialists be involved in the patient's care. However, continuity with one physician caring for the survivor adds greatly to the security of patient and family.
5. Monitoring the effect of cancer and treatment on the patient's ability to attain age-appropriate developmental tasks, especially in children and adolescents, with early referral for rehabilitation. This may entail neurological, endocrinological and psychological evaluation to arrive at a diagnosis and to introduce remediation.
6. Psychological intervention for significant anxiety and depression should be considered *early* to prevent more severe problems.
7. Evaluation of family interaction for possible impact of the stress on other family members, and to recognise maladaptation patterns.
8. "Veteran" patient support should be encouraged. The psychological gains from discussion with others who have the same neoplasm and who have experienced similar treatment is invaluable. At Memorial Sloan-Kettering a centre for survivors offers peer counselling, professional consultation and legal advice.

REFERENCES

1 Tross S and Holland JC: Psychological sequelae in cancer survivors. In: Massie MJ and Holland JC (eds) Handbook of Psychooncology: Psychological Care of the Cancer Patient. Oxford University Press, New York 1989

Screening for Breast Cancer

Peter Maguire

Cancer Research Campaign, Psychological Medicine Group, Christie Hospital, Manchester M20 9BX, United Kingdom

Screening for breast cancer has been or is being introduced within several European and Scandinavian countries. Its introduction is based on the assumption that tumours will be detected earlier and the length of survival increased. It has also been assumed that early diagnosis by screening will improve psychological adaptation in two ways. Firstly, women will feel more confident about their prognosis. Secondly, they will have more treatment options, for example, mastectomy versus wide local excision plus radiotherapy. Yet, there is still no firm evidence to support these assumptions about the favourable impact of screening on psychological adjustment to cancer.

Most women who notice that they have a lump, dimpling of the skin or nipple discharge, realise that it could be due to cancer. This forwarning helps them adapt when their fears are confirmed by subsequent examination and investigation. In contrast, most women attend for screening believing, in the absence of signs or symptoms, that they are free of cancer. The news that they have cancer must come as an unexpected shock and so may be harder to adapt to. Moreover, it may fuel fears that, if the cancer recurs, it will also be occult and there will be nothing they can do to ensure early intervention. So, it could well be that levels of distress will be higher and remain so in those with screen-detected cancers compared with those whose cancers are symptomatic.

Offering choice of treatment to some women appears to facilitate adaptation in the short term. But what about those other women who still wish to leave it to the doctor to decide on the best option? Does exercising choice enhance or hinder adaptation if the cancer recurs?

These are key questions which screening programmes need to address seriously and soon. Given the small numbers of screen-detected cancers within each centre, a multicentre collaborative study would appear to be the best solution.

Training in Psychosocial Oncology

Peter Maguire [1], Darius Razavi [2] and Robert Zittoun [3]

1 Cancer Research Campaign, Psychological Medicine Group, Christie Hospital, Manchester M20 9BX, United Kingdom
2 Service de Médecine et Laboratoire d'Investigation, Clinique H. Tagnon (Unité de Psycho-Oncologie), Institut Jules Bordet, Centre des Tumeurs de l'Université Libre de Bruxelles, 1 rue Héger Bordet, 1000 Brussels, Belgium
3 Service d'Hématologie, Hôtel Dieu, 1, Place du Parvis Notre Dame, 75181 Paris Cedex 04, France

If the psychological and social care of patients with cancer is to be of a uniformly good standard, those involved in cancer care must be better trained in basic interviewing, assessment and counselling skills. But there are not enough "experts" to provide this training. Therefore, training of key personnel in the required teaching methods is a priority. This area of training in particular and the field of psychosocial oncology in general should be rooted in solid research findings rather than in personal conjecture and belief. However, there are few formal opportunities for people to learn the relevant research methodology. This chapter will review some current initiatives in providing training in these aspects of psychosocial oncology.

Counselling

Few doctors and nurses involved in cancer care receive any formal training in basic interviewing, assessment and counselling skills. Nor do many of those nurses and social workers who take on specialist roles (such as breast cancer care, stoma care, care of children with cancer, or chemotherapy) obtain adequate training in these skills. Even if they have some training in counselling before being out into their posts, this is usually limited to non-directive methods like listening and reflecting. While such methods are of value in certain situations, they can be counter-productive in patients with cancer, as the following example illustrates.

Specialist nurse	How are you feeling now?
Patient (dying of cancer)	Depressed.
Specialist nurse	Depressed?
Patient	Yes, very depressed.
Specialist nurse	Very depressed.
Patient	Yes, very.

This led to a long silence during which the patient became increasingly withdrawn and depressed. The nurse did not know what to do next. Her training in counselling had not included advice about how to help patients talk more actively about such feelings and express them in a way which helped alleviate the worst of the depression.

While many courses for nurses wishing to specialise in oncology or specific aspects of cancer care claim to include training in counselling, this is rare in reality. Inputs on psychological assessment and counselling are few and usually didactic in form. Thus, a 3-month course in stoma care may include only 1 day on any aspect of counselling. Consequently, many involved in cancer care find they prefer to focus on practical and technical tasks, and distance themselves from psychological and social concerns. For example, in terminal care adequate pain control is vital but concern with pain control can become an effective distancing tactic [1]. Fortunately, attempts are being made to remedy these deficiencies.

Solutions

Basic Training

Medical, nursing and social work curricula are already full. But some room must be found for formal training in basic interviewing skills. These should include: the ability to acknowledge, clarify and organise key verbal and non-verbal cues that patients and relatives give about their problems; control (the ability to maintain the focus of the interview and help patients and relatives stick to the point without alienating them); precision (obtaining precise information, e.g., an exact date of a bereavement versus a vague date, since this encourages accurate recall and helps the relative or patient recall and express the associated feelings); the exploration of emotionally-loaded areas (e.g., worry about the future or the impact of illness on a personal relationship) in a way which is helpful and not too painful; and the use of open ("How are you feeling?") and directive questions ("How did you feel about having a stoma?"). For these skills are all associated with the better recognition of psychosocial problems [2] and those who use them are perceived as more empathic and understanding compared with those who do not.

These skills can only be improved through the provision of detailed handouts and videotapes which make the methods explicit, practice of the skills, recording and audio and videotape feedback of performance [3].

An increasing number of medical, nursing and social work schools are including this feedback training, although the overall number is still few. It is worth doing since the gains appear to persist over time [4], but it must be conducted by teachers who understand the skills being taught and can help students identify first their strengths and then their weakness. Basic training in medicine, nursing, or social work also includes a psychiatry attachment so that knowledge is gained about normal versus abnormal reactions, the range of possible interventions and indications for their use. This will facilitate basic interviewing and assessment.

Postbasic Training

A common response to deficiencies in basic training has been for teaching centres to mount study days on topics such as "talking with cancer patients", "counselling cancer patients", or "helping the bereaved". These may be aimed at one professional group or be multidisciplinary. There is a growing and welcome shift from lectures by experts to the use of videotapes to demonstrate key skills and small group work where these tapes can be discussed and particular skills practised in role play. Small group work can also be used to help participants identify areas of counselling which they would like help with. If study days lead some people to seek more training, they are worthwhile. But the idea that study days are a solution in themselves still receives much, albeit misguided, support. For those stimulated to seek more training, what is available?

Short workshops

Some initiatives have been taken to mount workshops whose aim is to help foster the development of counselling skills in those involved in cancer care. For example, two cancer charities, the Cancer Research Campaign and Help the Hospices, have supported 3 to 5-day workshops for doctors, nurses, social workers and chaplains. These workshops are residential and are held away from the workplace to facilitate sharing and learning. They are limited to a maximum of 20 participants.

They begin with participants meeting in two small groups to decide their agenda, that is, which particular assessment and counselling situations they feel they need help with as a result of their professional experience. Videotapes are then shown of a method of basic assessment and discussed. In this way, the areas that should be covered and the skills that should be used are made explicit. The participants then break into two small groups to practise, under the guidance of an experienced tutor, basic assessment and those counselling situations they placed high on their agenda [5]. They practise in carefully structured role play exercises, which are

structured to minimise the risk that participants will feel threatened, humiliated and deskilled.
Participants are instructed that when they comment on how the role play is going, they must emphasise all the perceived strengths first before any criticisms are made. When they make a criticism they must try to suggest an alternative strategy. The person attempting the assessment or counselling task is told that he must ask for time out if he feels he is stuck and should do this as soon as he feels stuck. The group members will then be asked to suggest what strategies might be used next. These can then be tested out in further role play. The person attempting the task then learns which of the offered strategies work best. The tutor should resist offering a solution unless the group fails to solve the problem.
A common criticism of role play is that it lacks realism. This is true if participants are assigned roles as patients or relatives which have little salience for them. In contrast, asking those who volunteered a task for the initial agenda like "dealing with anger", to play the part of the angry patient or relative they had difficulty with in real life, ensures it will be a realistic portrayal. It also gives them useful insights into how the patient or relative felt [5].
Problems which are most commonly practised in role play include basic assessment, breaking bad news, coping with a patient who has been lied to about his prognosis, handling difficult questions, dealing with anger, challenging denial, facing relatives after they have experienced a sudden unexpected death, breaking collusion and establishing a dialogue with a withdrawn patient. They are practised in order of increasing difficulty. To practise the most difficult situations first would cause the experienced participants to feel deskilled and angry. This risk of deskilling is also reduced by asking participants to stay within the brief developed out of the participant's experience by the tutor, and to avoid making it more difficult. If the role player deviates from the brief, or the assessor/counsellor gets stuck but does not call time out, the tutor intervenes.
As participants progress through the workshops, they become concerned about how they can apply their new skills within their own work and still survive emotionally. Therefore, a session is devoted to the identification and discussion of strategies that facilitate survival.

Follow Up

As with any teaching, there is a danger that short-term gains in skills are not maintained over time. Therefore, follow-up workshops are held 6 months later to consolidate learning and discuss any difficulties that have been encountered in attempting to apply the skills. Participants then practise more advanced counselling tasks. A scientific study is under way to evaluate which of the skills being taught are acquired and maintained over time. Preliminary analysis of participants' consultations with simulated patients immediately before and after the first workshops suggests there are significant gains in skills. The assessment of consultations immediately before the follow-up workshops will indicate if these skills are maintained.

Short Courses

In one study, small groups of health professionals were offered or asked to attend short courses on caring for the terminally ill [6]. These were flexible in their timetabling to allow for attendance by busy medical and nursing personnel. Consequently, although the courses lasted a total of 12 hours, sessions lasted from 75 to 180 minutes and courses comprised 4,6,8, or 10 sessions. The aims were to develop a greater understanding of death and dying and foster more positive attitudes towards care of the dying. Training methods included role play, comparing experiences, discussion of cases and theoretical concepts. The courses were led by psychologists and/or psychiatrists.
To assess their impact, each participant was asked to complete a semantic differential questionnaire [6] before and after the courses. A control group was assessed similarly. Those with negative attitudes before training showed most positive change in their attitudes. Whether participants were self-selected or selected did not affect change in attitudes. Self-regard and attitudes to the physician-patient relationship changed most. It is not yet known if gains in attitude are parallelled by changes in skill or maintained over time. But it demonstrates that personnel from a wide number of hospitals can be reached in this way.

Focussed Training

The workshops and short courses described cover a wide range of skills. Training might be more effective if it focussed on more limited objectives and reached more personnel within a shorter time period. One study focussed on the teaching of basic interviewing and assessment skills [7]. Ninety-six health workers and district nurses within two health districts were randomised to four training conditions: being taught the skills required; the areas to cover; both coverage and skills; and no training (control). Coverage and skills were first demonstrated by videotape. Participants then received audio feedback on practice interviews within small groups. Assessments were based on an analysis of recordings of assessment interviews conducted before and after showing the videotapes and after feedback training.

All subjects exhibited a low level of the required skills before training. All those receiving training showed significant improvements compared with the control group. Those taught both skills and coverage improved most. The use of the demonstration videotapes had a considerable and positive impact on skills. But there was a difference in outcome according to the area of assessment covered. Most improvement was evident in physical aspects such as the physical limitations caused by the cancer and the complications of treatment. While psychological assessment improved significantly from a statistical viewpoint, the level of psychological assessment after training was barely adequate.

The nurses admitted that they were still reluctant to cover psychological and social aspects in any depth. They had little confidence that the general practitioner would heed any feedback about psychological and social morbidity. They believed that they would be criticised by their nursing managers for "talking and not doing". They already had enough problems to contend with without looking for additional problems in patients with cancer and their relatives. So, any attempts at training must pay more attention to these contextual issues and to the affective domain of learning. For, although these nurses were committed to improving patient care, they did not see psychological care of cancer patients as important when judged against their other priorities such as care of young children and the elderly.

Training at Work

Workshops, short courses and focussed training are usually held away from the workplace. An alternative is to carry out the training within the working environment. For example, nurses on a surgical ward were given feedback training in interviewing and assessment skills by an experienced nurse teacher [8]. The aim was to improve their ability to assess the needs of patients with breast cancer. Many skills improved significantly although, as with the district nurses and health visitors, improvement was most marked in assessment of physical aspects. However, with ongoing supervision and support, they further improved and maintained their ability to recognise psychological and social morbidity and report this to the surgeons. Importantly, they claimed that they gained greater enrichment from their work.

In conclusion, it should be possible to offer such training to staff within each ward, outpatient and care area of a cancer hospital in turn, providing a suitable tutor is available. While nurses respond to this approach, doctors may be less receptive. Studies are needed to determine if doctors are prepared to participate.

Maintaining Skills

For those who attend workshops or short courses, a key question is how best to help them maintain and apply their learning over time. Two solutions are being attempted, the use of peripatetic teachers and distance learning. The peripatetic teacher follows up groups of participants according to their geographical location and helps them apply and continue their learning. Distance learning requires participants to practise particular assessment and counselling tasks, record their attempts using a tape recorder, and send the resultant tape to one of the workshop or course tutors for feedback. The effectiveness of these methods in helping maintain and further develop skills has still to be evaluated.

They might be especially effective if each cancer centre or hospital sent at least two people to a workshop or course for they could support each other in this further learning.

Long Courses

Some cancer centres have introduced full-time courses of several weeks' duration which aim to equip specialist nurses both in technical aspects and counselling skills. They seek to achieve this by training within the course and subsequent supervision of practice. This is a welcome development but it requires objective evaluation.

Such courses are few and doctors, nurses and social workers may turn, instead, to more general courses in counselling which require between several months' full attendance or up to 2 years' part-time attendance. These are usually offered by Universities or other higher education institutions and result in the award of a counselling certificate or diploma.

Conclusion

Longer formal courses of 3-6 months' duration are needed in addition to short workshops and courses to ensure that those who wish to take on specific assessment and counselling roles within cancer care are properly trained. Such courses should result in the award of a certificate or diploma and include supervision of counselling by audio or videotape recording and feedback.

Teaching

If training in assessment and counselling is to be improved, more teachers will be needed. Those cancer specialists, psychiatrists, psychologists, specialist nurses and social workers who are already committed to improving psychological and social care are a valuable resource, but most will require training in the relevant teaching methods.

They will be more effective in their teaching role if they first experience at first hand the methods they are intending to use [9]. If they then work in pairs to run workshops and courses, they are more likely to maintain a constructive momentum and be in a position to train others to teach. Such teacher training is still in its infancy but it is promising because of its potential "cascade" effect.

Research

Research into psychological and social aspects of oncology will only prosper if those interested in it have adequate opportunities for training in the relevant methodologies. But most research is still funded on a project basis. Therefore, research workers tend to come and go with the waxing and waning of projects. Fortunately, this problem has been recognised and several initiatives have been taken. For example, the Cancer Research Campaign has established two units within the United Kingdom which are focussing on longer term research. The Imperial Cancer Research Fund has established training posts for Senior Registrars in Psychiatry. The World Health Organisation has set up a unit concerned with quality-of-life measurement within clinical trials. Some major cancer centres, such as Memorial Sloan-Kettering in New York, have established academic departments of psychiatry. Others, like the Institut Jules Bordet, have departments of Psychosocial Oncology. These units can act as a resource for those wishing to obtain advice or training in research methodology and the EORTC and other agencies may be more prepared to fund training fellowships in this area in the near future. The EORTC has already encouraged the exchange of ideas and collaboration through its quality-of-life subgroup. Despite these initiatives, there is no formal training in research. Consequently, those who are interested have to rely on being appointed to a research project or programme and being trained within their costs. It is not surprising, then, that the standard of research is still too variable and that there is much unnecessary duplication of effort. The establishment of permanent Senior Research Fellows and training fellowships could help remedy these problems.

REFERENCES

1 Maguire P: Barriers to psychological care of the dying. Br Med J 1985 (291):1711-1713
2 Goldberg DP, Steele JJ, Smith C and Spivey L: Training family doctors to recognise psychiatric illness with increased accuracy. Lancet :521-523
3 Maguire P, Roe P, Goldberg D, Hyde C, Jones S and O'Dowd T: The value of feedback in teaching interviewing skills to medical students. Psychol Med 1978 (8):695-704
4 Maguire P, Fairbairn S and Fletcher C: Consultation skills of young doctors: 1. Benefits of feedback training in interviewing as students persist. Br Med J 1983 (292):1573-1578
5 Maguire P and Faulkner A: How to improve the counselling skills of doctors and nurses in cancer care. Br Med J 1988 (297):847-849
6 Razavi D, Delvaux N, Farvacques C and Robaye E: Immediate effectiveness of brief psychological training for health professionals dealing with terminally ill cancer patients: A controlled study. Soc Sci Med (27):369-375
7 Fairbairn S, Maguire P and Faulkner A: Training community nurses to assess and monitor patients with cancer. Report to the Cancer Research Campaign, London 1989
8 Faulkner A and Maguire P: Teaching ward nurses to monitor cancer patients. Clin Oncol 1984 (10):383-389
9 Naji SA, Maguire GP, Fairburn SA, Goldberg DP and Faragher EB: Training clinical teachers in psychiatry to teach interviewing skills. Med Educ 1986 (20):140-147

MIX
Papier aus verantwortungsvollen Quellen
Paper from responsible sources
FSC® C105338

If you have any concerns about our products,
you can contact us on
ProductSafety@springernature.com

In case Publisher is established outside the EU,
the EU authorized representative is:
Springer Nature Customer Service Center GmbH
Europaplatz 3, 69115 Heidelberg, Germany

Printed by Libri Plureos GmbH
in Hamburg, Germany